DISTRACTED

DISTRACTED

How Regulations Are Destroying the Practice of Medicine and Preventing True Health-Care Reform

MATTHEW HAHN, MD

Skyhorse Publishing

Visit our website at www.skyhorsepublishing.com.

10 9 8 7 6 5 4 3 2 1

Library of Congress Cataloging-in-Publication Data is available on file.

Cover design by Rain Saukas
Cover photograph: iStockphoto

Print ISBN: 978-1-5107-1511-0
Ebook ISBN: 978-1-5107-1513-4

Printed in the United States of America

For Bibi, who is most responsible for everything good in my life, and for Willa, for whom we want to make the world a better place.

For Russell. Our conversations over the years created the content of this book.

For my staff, Lindy, Amber, Tonya, and Mary, who give our patients exquisite care despite all the roadblocks.

And for our patients, and all patients, who all deserve the best care that is possible.

Contents

Introduction

I am a practicing family physician in a small rural town. In 2009, when most of my colleagues were leaving their practices to work for large health systems, I did the opposite, opening a small private practice with one other doctor. We brought along a small, extremely talented, and dedicated staff. My wife is the practice manager. Our practice's motto is "A new way to practice old-fashioned care."

And that's a good description of our practice. We try to see sick patients on the same day no matter what. We will see patients during the evening, on weekends when need be, and we even do house calls when necessary. We see all ages, and take care of all manner of chronic diseases. We get to know many of our patients like family, and we try to treat them even better.

And we embrace new technologies that revolutionize our ability to get our work done. I am also one of the founders of a small IT company that produced the electronic health record (EHR) software we use in our practice. It enables us to do the work of many with just a few.

We love what we do, and we live for it—it is our calling.

But the American health-care system is making it harder and harder to do what we love. And we fear that if things continue as they are now, it may someday soon become impossible.

In every practice I had previously worked, each much larger than mine today, I had been shielded from much of what went on. I couldn't see, and therefore didn't understand, many of the problems that were occurring. But with such a small office now, I get a bird's-eye view of everything. And my eyes have been opened. Unfortunately, much of what I see is horrifying.

I am witness to a tragedy. The once great American health-care system has fallen seriously ill. Millions of Americans are suffering the consequences.

Patients are literally dying at the hands of our health-care system. It takes as much of their money as possible first. Then it tries to kill them. Sometimes it actually succeeds. Think I'm exaggerating? As I sit writing these very words, I spy this headline from the *New York Times*: "Florida Man Says He Killed Sick Wife Because He Couldn't Afford Her Medicine, Sheriff Says."

That is American health care today—a system so sick that it often harms rather than heals. We have come to accept this, but it is completely unacceptable. And it could be easily fixed.

The symptoms of the illness are well known, and have been for a long time:

- Too many patients have limited or no access to medical care. Despite Obamacare, close to thirty million people in America still lack health insurance.
- American health care costs too much. According to a September 2015 report by the Kaiser Family Foundation/Health Research and Education Trust, annual premiums for employer-sponsored family health coverage have reached an astounding $17,545. In

July 2016, the US Department of Health and Human Services reported that per-person spending on health care in the United States had gone over $10,000, easily more than twice the amount spent in most of the world's other developed countries.

- American health care is poor-outcome health care. A 2014 survey by the Commonwealth Fund reported that "the United States health care system is the most expensive in the world (and) among the 11 nations studied in this report—the U.S. ranks last." And shockingly, a May 2016 article in the *British Medical Journal* reported that medical errors were the "third leading cause of death" in the United States.

Yet despite knowing the symptoms, and despite massive efforts to make things right, they are getting progressively worse.

And here is one of the biggest reasons why. More and more, doctors and nurses fight not against disease, but against a rule-crazed administrative system hell-bent on wasting their time and denying patients care. They are being driven away from and even out of patient care, forced to focus instead on compliance with an ever-expanding universe of pointless rules and harmful regulations devised by bureaucrats and administrators who have no idea what they are doing and have little regard for the consequences of their actions.

The practice of medicine, providing care to patients, has been shoved aside, replaced by a sea of distractions. There is less time for patient care, too many diversions during patient care, and no time to focus on improving care—only time to fill out newly required forms, to try to keep up and catch up using unusable computer systems, to learn and negotiate the insane workarounds necessary to obtain care in this system, and to collect more data—always more data—to satisfy the new health-care rule-makers.

While smaller practices like mine find this particularly challenging, we are not the only ones having trouble. The same problems are being experienced throughout the health-care system. My colleagues who have gone to work for larger practices and health systems complain of the same things. Their days, and often their nights as well, are spent struggling to keep up with the added distractions and increasing administrative demands.

A well-publicized study published in the September 6, 2016, issue of the *Annals of Internal Medicine* concluded, "For every hour physicians provide direct clinical face time to patients, nearly 2 additional hours is spent on EHR and desk work within the clinic day. Outside office hours, physicians spend another 1 to 2 hours of personal time each night doing additional computer and other clerical work."

It is a system that is not working for anyone. It is dangerous for patients and incredibly demoralizing for health-care professionals.

But seeing what is going on from my close-up vantage point, one that few physicians (and none of our policymakers or media) today are afforded, has given me a unique view of what is going on. And as I began to see the issues more clearly, I realized that the national conversation regarding health care in the United States was largely missing many of the most crucial points—the very issues that make or break our efforts to reform the system. It also became apparent that there is a much better way forward.

Distracted reveals these often-shocking details using real experiences from deep within our ailing health-care system. More importantly, based on the hard-learned lessons detailed in each chapter, *Distracted* offers simple, concrete, and commonsense solutions for each of these problems.

CHAPTER 1

Distracted

I f you want to learn what is wrong with the American health-care system, just follow any doctor or nurse (or any patient for that matter) for just a short time. It will soon become obvious. The following common scenario should make things clear.

A patient comes to the office or the hospital—that is, if he can afford to come at all. If he has no insurance (still common), or he has a hefty co-pay or a huge insurance deductible (which is becoming more common), he may avoid care altogether. But let's assume, for the sake of our story, that he gets past these common barriers.

The patient is greeted in the customary manner, "How are you going to pay for this?" Only after this question is answered satisfactorily can the clinical portion of the appointment commence.

The patient is taken to the exam room, and the doctor or nurse attempts to pull up his medical record on a computer in the corner. It is common to use computerized medical records today even though in some ways they are worse than the paper charts they replaced. They can be painfully expensive, often slow things down considerably, and are felt by many to be largely unusable in the throes of patient care. But the government has mandated their use, and there are substantial penalties for failing to comply. So, they are used.

But because of an Internet slowdown (many computerized medical records are Internet-based, so this often happens), there is a substantial delay, precious minutes, until the record comes up. If it happens to be one of the days when the system just isn't functioning, backup paper charts are used instead. The computerized system will have to be updated later, though, which will duplicate the work and double the amount of time spent filling out the chart.

To fill the awkward void created by these wait times, the doctor and the patient chitchat about how bad things are in the world, especially in health care.

When the patient's record is finally displayed, the doctor has to open and close multiple screens just to view basic medical information, which slows things down even further. It is also distracting, especially as the doctor attempts simultaneously to interact with the patient like he is a human being. This interaction is important because it allows the doctor to pick up important clues to what is wrong with the patient, but also because after the appointment, the patient will be filling out a government-mandated satisfaction survey that partly determines how much the doctor gets paid. Not surprisingly, staring incessantly at the computer screen rather than making eye contact with the patient often results in lower satisfaction scores.

Attempting to have a human interaction is made even more challenging by the fact that the computer, an old PC, is on a desk facing away from the patient, so to manage the computer and try to make eye contact with the patient now and then, the doctor twists her head around and around, like Linda Blair in *The Exorcist*. Talk about distracting!

While the patient discusses his medical history, the doctor's mind wanders, as it often tends to, to the incredibly complicated, but government-mandated, formula used to calculate how much should be charged for the appointment. As required, the doctor tries to keep count of how many problems the patient complains about, the number of questions that were discussed in relation to each of those problems, and even the number of body systems that were reviewed in each case. As the formula specifies, the more that is discussed, the more that can be charged for the appointment. The same goes for the physical exam—the more body parts examined, the more that can be charged, so the doctor tries to keep count of that, as well. Sometimes during computer slowdowns, the doctor fantasizes about a patient with an extra arm and an extra leg, and wonders how much she could charge for that (probably an arm and a leg).

I am not making this up, by the way. I realize this is hard to believe, but this is exactly how things are done.

So, based on what the doctor learns from the patient's history and physical exam, she attempts to clear her head of all the distractions and to formulate a plan of care. She appropriately surmises that some testing would be useful in helping to pinpoint the possible diagnoses. But getting the tests is easier said than done. First of all, the electronic health record's ordering system is a little quirky in that it requires that any tests be entered twice, which is annoying and time-consuming. Adding insult to injury, after the doctor finishes double entering the test orders, and twists her head around owl-style to explain the reason for the testing, the patient then says he would rather the doctor hold off on any testing. The patient explains that he has a high-deductible insurance policy, which means that he would have to pay for any tests, or almost any health care he receives for that matter, out of pocket. But after paying his exorbitant health insurance premiums, there is no money left for such things. Both the patient and the doctor again take a few moments to complain bitterly about all of this. This extra time complaining has become such a regular part of many appointments that the doctor has even daydreamed about a system where she could bill for complaining. In her dream, she gets rich quickly and then retires!

When they both finish complaining, the doctor also remembers that Medicare and many insurance companies are now monitoring how many tests and treatments she orders and comparing the cost of her medical care to that of other doctors. Beginning in 2019, there will be financial penalties if her care exceeds the average, one of the horrors contained in the new government payment reform plan, the Medicare Access and CHIP Reauthorization Act (known better by its abbreviation, MACRA). Unfortunately, how these penalties will get calculated is not particularly clear. Nor is it clear what the doctor is supposed to do if she just happens to have a lot of sick patients that require expensive care. But it is clear that she doesn't want to be penalized, so, the doctor thinks, to hell with clinical relevance and the best interests of the patient. With all of those things getting in the way, she is not ordering any testing.

Since the doctor won't have the benefit of any tests to confirm her suspicions, she just makes her best guess at the diagnosis that is most likely. But she also takes the time to explain to the patient that she just might be missing the far more deadly (though somewhat less likely) diagnosis she might have found had she been able to get any testing. This understandably upsets the patient, who requests some Valium because he is so distressed. With the threat of a negative patient satisfaction score looming over her head, the doctor gives him the Valium.

The doctor also prescribes a medicine based on her test-free diagnostic guess. She knows that this is not an optimal way to decide on something as important as a patient's medical care, but her hands are tied. The doctor sends the prescription, which is a commonly used generic medication, to the patient's pharmacy, but then receives a call from them to say that this medication, which she's been prescribing for many years, is no longer available unless she first obtains prior authorization from the patient's insurance company. She gets on the phone and waits for ten (unpaid) minutes to get the authorization, but then gets cut off without completing the process.

On a completely separate, but very important, matter, the doctor also happens to note that the patient's blood pressure is quite high (she assumes hers is too at this point). Even though the patient did not come in to discuss this issue, the doctor decides that it's too important to ignore. When she brings this to the patient's attention, he admits that he stopped his blood pressure pills because he received a notice that the medication, which he had been taking for the last ten years, was no longer on his formulary, and he couldn't afford to pay for it on his own.

The patient also relates that he is so stressed and tired from working two jobs that he doesn't feel he has time to exercise or eat well. He gets home late and eats to comfort himself, he says. He has gained ten pounds since his last visit.

This is a problem for the patient, obviously, but it's a problem for the doctor now as well, because the government has started collecting and compiling statistics that rate the quality of a doctor's care based on such things as the blood pressures of patients treated for hypertension (high blood pressure). Beginning in 2019, as part of the previously mentioned MACRA program, there will be financial penalties for low quality ratings.

So the government assesses penalties if the patient's blood pressure is not well controlled, even though the patient's insurance doesn't cover his blood pressure medication. The doctor and the patient are caught between a rock (the government) and a hard place (the insurance company).

With so many factors working against them, and especially in light of these looming penalties, the doctor begins to think it would just be better if the patient (whom she has been seeing for years) went somewhere else for his medical care. Why should she be penalized when there are so many factors entirely beyond her control that keep her from adequately caring for such patients? But wait, there's more.

At the end of the appointment, the doctor remembers that government regulations mandate that she prepare and print out a summary of the visit for the patient. And then she has to click a box to validate that she did this.

She is also forced by government mandate to discuss (and check the box that indicates her having done this) that her practice now offers an online portal where the patient can access his medical records and communicate with the clinical staff. As dumb as it sounds—and as dumb as she feels doing it—she also encourages the patient to go to the portal and drop her a line in the next few days, because she needs to get a certain percentage of patients to do that in order to satisfy another government quality measure. So, throughout her already-too-busy day, she now receives and has to respond to any number of patient emails that go something like this: "Hi doc, I'm writing you an email like you asked. How's it going?"

And finally, the doctor prints out an educational handout for the patient regarding the guessed-at diagnosis, and then clicks yet another box documenting that she did this because, you guessed it, giving patients educational materials is government mandated, and there are penalties for not doing it.

The doctor has always been a proud American, but in her quieter moments she now often finds herself fantasizing about what she might do to the government bureaucrats who create all these idiotic mandates.

Frustrated, distracted, and now running late for her next appointment, the doctor decides to write up her notes later that night, or maybe early the next morning, because the computer system is just too slow to do it while she is seeing the patient. She knows that she will probably forget important points by the time she gets to it, especially considering all of the distractions she has encountered. She and her colleagues now spend hours after they are done seeing patients trying to catch up on the computer, and this is beginning to take a terrible toll. But that's just how it is these days.

I will stop there. Do you get a sense from this vignette what might be wrong with the American health-care system? This type of scenario plays out all day, every day, and it makes doctors just want to give up and throw in the towel. It makes highly trained professionals who once loved taking care of patients think about quitting. It is a situation that is demoralizing for both patients and their doctors. And occasionally, it just happens to kill a patient or two.

As the scenario plainly demonstrates, medical professionals are increasingly distracted by a combination of overly burdensome and needlessly complicated government regulation and a health insurance industry that systematically denies necessary medical care.

I am not a traditionalist. There was no golden era of medicine to which I think we need to return. Taking care of patients has always been challenging and it always will be, even under the best of circumstances. But years ago the process was a hell of a lot more straightforward than it is today. I am not advocating a return to the past, but what is happening today is unacceptable. We need a better way forward. Our lives may depend on it. The lives of our family members may depend on it.

The Real Devil Is in the Details

Unfortunately, the public discourse regarding health care in America barely scratches the surface of what is really wrong. So much crucial detail is missing that it is a conversation with very little true value.

It touches on the "big picture" only—the biggest trends, the biggest scares, the largest profits and losses—but it is so far removed from the reality of what is happening that it is a distorted and inaccurate view. And discussions regarding "health-care reform" focus primarily on how payment for health care in the US should be organized. Too much else that is crucial to the conversation is not being discussed. The real devil, the real value, and the real solutions lie deeper within—within details with which too few are familiar, both inside and outside of the health-care profession.

Knowing these details is essential for a number of reasons. First of all, without an accurate grasp of the problems that plague health care, it is unlikely we will fix things properly. Just as important, these details, which are largely absent from typical discussions regarding health-care reform, are actually the key to its success or failure. No matter which popular reform model we ultimately select—multi-payer, single-payer, for-profit, or not-for-profit—it is the details we will discuss in *Distracted* that make or break each of these approaches.

And finally, if you do not know the details, and the devil within them, it is easy to believe government bureaucrats, who say they understand the problems and have a plan to make things right. On the surface, their solutions often sound plausible. In reality, they themselves are the problem.

The bureaucratic narrative goes something like this. The problem is that we have traditionally paid for health care based solely on volume (a fee-for-service system), which rewards quantity but ignores quality. This approach leads to costly, low-quality health care. And there is certainly some truth to that explanation. Their solution is to create a system that pays for quality and performance (referred to as pay-for-performance or a value-based payment system) rather than volume. And furthermore, they say that we can use health information technology to collect data that measures performance in relation to objective clinical standards, and then tie financial incentives and penalties to the results. It sounds like a reasonable approach.

And the fact is that this could be part of an effective approach, but in the details—the methods they use, the implementation, and the execution—things go terribly wrong. *Distracted* tells the story of those often-bizarre details but also offers workable solutions.

The details reveal a number of recurring themes:

- It is not really "health care" that is failing—what is failing is the *administration* of health care. If you want a more accurate picture of what is wrong with the American health-care system, it is necessary to distinguish *health care*, referring to the doctors, the nurses, the diagnostics, the treatments, and the patients (let's not forget them), from *health-care administration*—referring to the government bureaucrats and health insurance executives and administrators, the bureaucracy they have created, and their heavy-handed and ineffective methods. That is the root of what is sickening our health-care system.
- A large and growing aspect of Americans' health care is dictated not by doctors and nurses, and certainly not by patients themselves, but by government bureaucrats and insurance-company administrators who have unlimited power and exert unfettered control over many aspects of our health and medical decision-making. But their overriding concern is money. Patient care and patients, for that matter, are lower down on their list of priorities.
- These bureaucrats' weapon of choice—an abundance of overly prescriptive rules and intrusive regulations, each tied to its own burdensome documentation requirements and performance measures—does more to impede true health-care reform than to promote it. In their misguided attempts to control what

happens in hospitals and doctors' offices, bureaucrats, people who do not take care of patients themselves, have created multiple layers of confusing rules and complicated programs whose chief effect is to distract those who do. Their efforts have had little appreciable effect on the quality and costs of medical care. And yet, with complete control and accountable to no one but themselves, they continue with more of the same. It is becoming an increasingly vicious cycle.

- Without the basic building blocks of health-system success—a simple, functional payment system; affordable, usable computer systems that communicate with one another and that are available to all physicians; and the elimination of the common barriers that keep patients from the care they need—any efforts to reform our health-care system are doomed to continued failure.

The government and the private sector share equally in the blame for what is wrong.

In an article titled "The Rise of the Hospital Administrator," from a blog called *The Doctor Weighs In*, Kevin Campbell, MD, writes, "In the past, physicians were responsible for both the business and practice of medicine. While administrative personnel played an important and complementary role in practice and hospital management, physicians were the cornerstone." By contrast, however, today "the leadership structure in medicine is now an entirely foreign landscape. Administrators dominate medical practices today. According to the *New York Times*, their salaries are responsible for a high percentage of medical costs. While the numbers of physicians that are entering the workforce have trended toward a constant number (with little or no growth) the numbers of administrators has risen nearly 3,000 percent over the last 30 years."

But these bureaucrats, the emperors who oversee modern health care, are wearing no clothes. Yet with totalitarian power to do so, they continue to heap more confusing and ineffective rules and regulations onto the burning pile.

Time Is of the Essence

Government bureaucrats, having ruined teaching through overregulation, are turning their attention more and more toward health care, their next victim. And insurance companies are tightening their grip on a captive population.

And good, caring doctors and nurses are leaving health care out of frustration. The physician and nursing shortages that are already gripping much of the nation will become much worse.

And patients are suffering at the hands of the system. We must demand better. Our lives depend on it.

CHAPTER 2

Getting Paid—Part 1:
You're Not Gonna Believe
How Your Bill Is Calculated

oney—it is the heart, to make somewhat of a pun, even the lifeblood, of our medical system, which is a shame because few of us have enough to pay for even a fraction of our health-care costs. But money, more than anything else, drives health care in the United States. I was naïve enough early in my career to think it was the other way around. I even told my staff, "We take excellent care of our patients. The money will follow." Now that I am a grizzled veteran of almost twenty years of health-care battles, I know that's not how it works. To make it through the day, we still cling to the notion that patients come first, but all day long, the system hammers home the message that it is really about the money. Patients, patient care, and doctors, as well, are somewhere lower on the list.

It is ironic, given such priorities, that we make the process of getting paid in health care so damn difficult. But that is just what we do. For physicians, getting paid represents a colossal hassle, an insane waste of time and energy. I am not talking, or complaining, about how much physicians are paid. That is another issue entirely. What I am referring to is the actual process by which physicians are paid.

In short, the payment system in American health care stinks. It is so bizarrely convoluted that it is unlikely that any one person knows or understands all of it. It has spawned an entire industry—the medical billing industry—that is necessary just to administer it. It even has its own college-level degrees. The system creates waste, encourages fraud, increases health-care costs, and in and of itself stands between patients and the care they need. As you will soon learn, it is also a great source of distraction to doctors and nurses. But the topic also marks a fitting place to start our journey in *Distracted* because difficulties getting paid are typically the first and worst nonmedical problem most health-care professionals come up against.

And it's been terrible for a long time. Much of the system in place today was instituted in 1995 or earlier. We complained bitterly back then, but we had no idea how good we actually had it. Aside from problems getting paid, at that time everything else more or less seemed to work, allowing us to actually focus on how best to care for our patients. We have so many more things we worry about today, it's disturbing. But since getting paid was our first problem, and many still consider it the worst problem, it will be our first topic. And if we can fix it, maybe we can fix the rest, as well. That's the spirit, right?

In "Getting Paid—Part 1," we discuss the ridiculous way we calculate a bill for a visit to a doctor's office. Then, in "Getting Paid—Part 2," we deal with the ridiculous way that the bill gets paid (or not).

You Must Be Kidding Me

I remember quite well the moment I was first introduced to "getting paid" for my doctoring services. It had not come up during the long four years of medical school. Believe it or not, the topic was almost entirely ignored. In fact, we were given the distinct impression that we were above such mundane and distasteful things.

Getting paid was first mentioned during the very early days of my family medicine residency. In residency, you are a full-fledged doctor, having graduated medical school, and therefore, have an "MD" attached to the end of your name. But let's just say there is a lot left to learn. It is tradition for residency to begin in July, and as many people know, you should try not to get sick that time of year because of this.

The first few days of residency were enjoyable because we weren't actually seeing patients. We were given a first-class orientation instead. We trained to run emergency resuscitations, were fitted with special respirators, and did other seemingly heroic things, such as getting special badges, filling out forms, and getting fed. I really liked those early days. I wore my crisp new long white coat like a superhero's cape. I was finally a real doctor, with all the esteem that went along with the title but, at least that first week, no real responsibilities to tarnish the glow. That was okay with me because I was thrilled to be a doctor (my mom was thrilled even more), but at the time, I was scared out of my mind about things like actually having to see patients and all of the other things that patients expected from real doctors—like knowing what they were doing.

As part of our preparations that first week, we also sat down with Dr. Andre Lijoi, the faculty member whose task it was to educate us about getting paid. It felt like we were talking to Dad about the birds and the bees. On the plus side, Dr. Lijoi had a gift for us (we were getting lots of free things that week). He gave us each our very own copies of the "Pocket Guide to the 1997 E/M Documentation Guidelines." This was a laminated card that would serve as our getting-paid cheat sheet. Resident physicians love cheat sheets. Our pockets were stuffed with all manner of them. "E/M" stands for "Evaluation and Management"—these guidelines outlined the complicated rules and the multitudes of specialized codes used in calculating the level of payment for a medical visit—in other words, how much you get paid. Dr. Lijoi explained that in order to be paid, a physician must submit, at a minimum, an E/M level of payment code, paired with a diagnosis code, to a patient's insurance company. On the negative side, what Dr. Lijoi told us that day was exceedingly boring and largely incomprehensible. And now I will attempt to explain this boring and incomprehensible topic to you.

Dr. Lijoi first explained that there was one set of E/M codes for new patients and another for established patients who had been to your office before. That wasn't so bad. I could grasp that. He went on to explain that the way we calculated the level of the visit for a new patient was slightly different from the way we did it for an established one. So things were getting just a little more complicated. But the bottom dropped out completely when he informed us that the level of visit depended on things like whether the history we obtained from the patient was "Problem Focused (PF)," "Expanded Problem Focused (EPF)," or "Detailed (D)." That is officially where I became lost. I am still trying to find my way.

You may want to get some coffee before reading this next paragraph, but try to bear with me. Dr. Lijoi explained that determining whether your patient's history was Problem Focused, Expanded Problem Focused, or Detailed required that you satisfy three out of three criteria from the history of present illness (HPI), the review of systems (ROS), and the past/family/social history (PFSH). To get a

Problem Focused history, you just needed between one and three elements from the history of the present illness. For an Expanded Problem Focused history, you needed one to three elements from the HPI as well as one body system from the ROS. For the Detailed history, which by the way, gets you a bunch more money, you needed more than three elements from the HPI, between two and nine elements from the ROS, and one element from the PFSH. At this point, you might begin to need an ibuprofen for your head-ache—but a drink might be better. By the way, I am not making this up.

But, believe it or not, that was just the first step in calculating the level-of-visit code. Dr. Lijoi explained that there were two additional calculations that needed to be performed. I will not bore you with those now, but I will bore you with them later.

My initial reaction that day was utter denial. I am not kidding. I assumed Dr. Lijoi must have been confused. I refused to believe that this was how it was done. Anyway, it didn't really matter, I reasoned, because there was no way I would ever comprehend such an insane system. My eyes glazed over, and my mind wandered back to the more heroic aspects of my new job, like the fact that my new coat had my name inscribed in red on the pocket. I understand now why the topic of payment had never been raised during medical school. We would have quit!

At the time, I could not grasp how I could be expected to both see patients *and* do this ridiculous calculation at the same time. We were actually given an entire hour to see a patient in those early days of our training (most practicing family physicians are trained, even today, to eventually be able to see patients in fifteen-minute time slots). My initial estimate was that the level-of-visit calculation would take me another hour or two, so this would have meant that I could see maybe one or two patients in a typical day. I was pretty sure that wasn't going to pay the bills.

Near the end of our session, Dr. Lijoi also introduced us to something called the "superbill," a complicated paper billing form that we were required to fill out after each patient appointment. The superbill is used to transmit billing information for the appointment to the office's billing staff. On the superbill, we wrote the diagnosis, checked off any tests or procedures we had performed (so that we could get paid for them), and indicated the dreaded E/M level-of-visit code, which implied that we had spent the extra hour actually trying to calculate it.

As an aside—there has been a superbill used in every practice I have worked since, though now the one I use is computerized. No one has ever explained to me why we call it a "superbill" and not just a "bill." What makes it so super? I don't complain about things like this, though, because adding the word "super" for no particular reason is a cool thing to do, and mine is a profession that often lacks cool.

But, quite obviously, I digress. Dr. Lijoi soldiered on till the blessed end of the session. Sensing that our minds were elsewhere, he encouraged us, "Don't worry, you'll pick it up as you go along." We were naïve and energetic, so we set about the imposing task. It is now about twenty years later, and as I said, I am still trying.

How Much Work Does a Doctor Do?

So, what are these E/M Documentation Guidelines, and why have we been afflicted with them? They are a mandatory system developed by the Centers for Medicare and Medicaid Services—CMS, which was then known as the Health Care Financing Administration (HCFA)—the government agency charged with administering large aspects of the US health-care system. The Evaluation and Management Documentation Guidelines specify how we calculate the amount we can bill for the work and the thought that go into a medical appointment. All doctors and other health-care practitioners must use these guidelines. Unfortunately, they are bizarrely complicated.

Apparently, prior to 1995, the E/M guidelines were somewhat vague. The guidelines were so vague that when I have queried my more experienced (by that I mean older) physician colleagues how they calculated the level of a visit prior to 1995, they all rubbed their heads and said something like, "I can barely remember." Suffice to say that prior to 1995, doctors essentially guesstimated how much they billed for an appointment.

But this troubled CMS for a number of reasons. First of all, CMS was not getting what they felt to be accurate data about the work that physicians were performing. Also, there was no effective way to know if physicians were "up-coding," billing for a higher level of service than they had actually performed. These were valid concerns. And it was becoming of increasing concern to CMS at that time because health-care costs for the nation were beginning to skyrocket (back then health care accounted for a paltry 8 percent of the gross domestic product; today that number is about 18 percent).

Another valid concern was that physicians' documentation of their work, their chart notes, often left a lot to be desired. Chart notes were often sparse, sometimes just a series of illegible abbreviations and shorthand. Incomplete and inconsistent chart notes encouraged errors. Prior to the introduction of the new guidelines, CMS had no way to influence what went into the physician's note, and this troubled them, understandably.

And so, in 1995, CMS introduced what it felt to be an elegant solution. They constructed a billing algorithm that matched the desired format of a physician's clinical note. It's the type of idea that on paper, or in a bureaucrat's office, seems sensible. But what it demonstrates is a pattern that we will see repeatedly throughout *Distracted*—a real and important problem that is addressed in a manner that seems conceptually sound, but that, in its real-life implementation, is so complicated and becomes so burdensome that it undoes its original intent. The old problems are replaced by new ones that make us nostalgic for the old ones.

But, as I have said, to understand the real devil, one must know the details. And here are the first of those details. I apologize in advance. What you need to know, first of all, is that all physicians are taught a very detailed format that they use to document what occurs during a patient appointment. It is a wonderful system referred to as the "SOAP" note. "SOAP" stands for:

- Subjective
- Objective
- Assessment
- Plan

Subjective refers to the patient's history, or their personal account of what is wrong with them. Objective refers to the data that a physician collects, such as the patient's vital signs, their physical exam findings, and the results of any testing done during the appointment. Assessment refers to the doctor's diagnosis, and might also include an explanation of their reasoning about such things. And then the Plan refers to the doctor's treatment of the patient, including such things as ordering testing, prescribing medications, or referring the patient for further care with another doctor.

Not to bore you too much, but it is important to understand a few more details. The Subjective portion of the note is classically divided into three sections:

- The chief complaint, a very brief statement of why the patient has come to the doctor

- The history of present illness (or HPI), which includes the following elements to describe a patient's complaint:
  - Duration of the symptom
  - Severity of the symptom
  - Location of pain (for a complaint of pain, an injury, or a rash)
  - Quality of the pain, such as sharp, dull, etc.
  - Context
  - What makes it better or worse
  - Treatments
  - Associated signs and symptoms
- The review of systems (ROS), which consists of questions used to refine the patient's complaint, typically categorized and assigned to the different body systems (i.e., the skin, the heart and vascular system, the lungs, etc.)

Then, the Objective (or physical exam) portion of the note is also typically categorized by body systems, and is usually presented roughly from head to toe (i.e., the neurologic system; ears, nose, and throat; heart; lungs; gastrointestinal system; etc.).

The significance of the SOAP note system cannot be overstated from a clinical perspective. At first glance, it may seem complicated, but in fact, it is an elegant system. It provides an effective organizational framework for almost all medical care, and is also the basis of a common language that all physicians speak. A well-constructed and documented SOAP note is the foundation of quality medical care. Medical students are drilled on this format until it becomes second nature. When I see a patient, I always look to my (or my colleagues') previous SOAP note(s), which leave a clear footprint of the care that was previously delivered. I think most clinicians would agree that the SOAP note format is a good one and that chart notes should be documented using it.

It is understandable, therefore, why CMS would want to link billing for a medical appointment to the SOAP note-charting system. The basic concept makes sense. The complexity and the work of a patient's appointment should be reflected in the amount of documentation included in a doctor's SOAP note. And the more work that is done, and the more documentation that is included, the higher the payment amount should be.

They Just Went Way Too Far

Here's the problem—and it is a very big problem. CMS constructed a billing formula based on the SOAP note format that is far more complicated than most actual SOAP notes. In fact, it is so much more complicated that, while medical students can learn the SOAP note format and begin to use it in a relatively short period of time, it actually takes college-level courses to learn E/M coding.

The E/M Documentation Guidelines are the perfection of bad. It is overkill on the scale of what we did to the American bison in the 1800s. It's as if, as a joke, they had a contest to see who could devise the worst system possible, one that would be guaranteed to be problematic, and even fail, and this was the winner. I have even wondered if someone really did propose the system as a joke, but then by mistake it caught on, and then no one had the guts to say anything. If I sound a little negative, it's because I am.

But let me explain. Remember that I promised to bore you more about the details of the E/M guidelines? This is when I do that, and once again, I apologize. After reading about this, I think you will understand one of the reasons that your physician might seem less than engaged in you and your care—in other words, why they might seem so distracted. It is because they are thinking about this rather than you.

But let's also put this into some necessary perspective. The level-of-visit algorithm I am about to describe is used to calculate how much a doctor can charge for an office visit, which, on average, amounts to about $75. It is hard to believe the amount of work and the number of steps that go into collecting a fee comparable to what you might pay for dinner at a restaurant.

But I will also let you in on a bit of a quandary I have in writing a book that focuses on bureaucracy and administration. It can be mind-numbingly boring. What I am about to describe is definitely mind-numbingly boring, and, therefore, I have struggled finding a balance between what might be readable and informative and what might make you throw the book (or your Kindle) into the fire. I hope I get it right. But I also go back to my central theses—that it is the administration of health care that is broken and that the real devil is in the details. And these details are what distinguishes a working health-care payment system from one that is so bad that it distracts doctors and endangers patients. And so, without further ado, here is the rest of how we calculate the amount we can charge for a doctor's appointment.

First of all, there a multitude of code sets from which to choose. As stated previously, there are separate sets of codes for a new patient's visit and for an established patient's subsequent appointments. There is also a set of codes for most problem-related office visits (such as an illness or injury, or a checkup for a chronic condition like high blood pressure), and then a completely separate set of codes (which have their own format) for preventive visits, like children's well-child checkups or adults' annual physicals (these are divvied up by age groups). There are *other* sets of codes for house calls, which I do from time to time, and for visits to other medical facilities, but let's keep this as simple as possible for now. I'm sure your eyes are glazing over with just these. Try to stay awake! Pinch yourself if need be.

New patient and the established patient office visits are then divided into five levels each:

- New patient codes: 99201, 99202, 99203, 99204, 99205
- Established patient codes: 99211, 99212, 99213, 99214, 99215

There are then strict criteria that define each of the five codes. To make things even more challenging, those criteria are slightly different for new and established patients. Is this starting to make sense yet?

Now try to follow me here (as Dr. Lijoi said, it gets easier—like when you're dead). For a new patient, calculating the level of visit entails satisfying the necessary documentation requirements for all three of the following, but for an established patient, the calculation requires satisfying only two of the three (doctor's choice which two):

1. History
2. Physical exam
3. Medical decision-making

Wake up, now. You can't be a doctor if you don't pick this up.

99211 to 99215 . . . Who's on First?

To make things easier then, let's just focus on the established patient codes. As I mentioned, you only need to satisfy two of the three criteria listed above.

First of all, there's the 99211. A 99211 is used for a visit that does not require the presence of a physician, like a visit with a nurse to check blood pressure. It has no specific documentation requirements, so it's an easy one. That was a good one to start with then, right?

Okay, now for 99212 to 99215. For fun, try to read this next section and digest it all, while you are also thinking about the last time you went to the doctor and everything that took place during that visit. In reality, that's exactly what doctors have to do—they focus on every patient from a clinical perspective, and at the same time, attempt to keep a running tally of the bill using the complex algorithm detailed below—it's not easy.

So, a 99212 code is used for an extremely simple visit, the type that often ends in my saying, "It's a mosquito bite." For a 99212, you need to document a chief complaint, and then two of three of the following: a history that includes a history of present illness (HPI) with one to three elements, no review of systems (ROS), and no review of past/family/social history (PFSH); an exam with one body system with between one and five individual elements; and straightforward medical decision-making. That was easy, right? It better be, because that's the simple one.

On to the 99213, which is the most common level-of-visit code we use. A 99213 is used for a simple illness or injury, or a checkup of one or two simple chronic illnesses. To code a 99213, you need to document a chief complaint, and then two of three of the following: a history with between one and three elements, a pertinent ROS, and no PFSH review; a physical exam with two to four body systems that includes a total of six to eleven individual elements; and low-complexity medical decision-making. I think they could bury Jimmy Hoffa in this calculation and no one would ever find him.

The 99214 is my favorite because it helps pay for my daughter's college far more than the 99213, but it doesn't get me audited like the 99215 would if I used it very often. Code 99214 is used for a more complicated illness or injury, or a checkup for three or more chronic illnesses. To code a 99214, you need a chief complaint (of course); and then two of three of the following: a history with at least four elements or at least three chronic diseases, a ROS that covers between two and nine body systems, and one element from the PFSH; a physical exam with five to seven body systems with a total of twelve or more individual elements; and moderate-complexity medical decision-making. And BINGO was his name-o.

And finally (*ka-ching*), there's code 99215, which is used for a very serious or complicated problem, one that might require treatment in the office or even calling an ambulance (or both). For a 99215, you need a chief complaint (but you know that by now); and then two of three of the following: a history with at least four elements or at least three chronic diseases, an ROS that covers at least ten body systems, and two elements from the PFSH; a comprehensive physical exam with at least eight body systems; and high-complexity medical decision-making, and, hopefully, a glass of decent scotch.

And then, for a 99216—oh, sorry, there is no 99216, I just kept going out of habit. But I have fantasized about a 99216 visit, and in my mind, it's real and it's spectacular.

See? I wasn't kidding, and I wasn't exaggerating. That's how we calculate how much we can get paid for a medical appointment, and it's a ridiculous way to do it.

As an aside—I would clarify what is meant by medical decision-making that is straightforward, low-complexity, moderate-complexity, or high-complexity, but I've never really been able to figure this out, and every time I try (like when I reviewed the material in preparation for this book), by the time I get through the criteria for the history and physical exam, I usually just give up.

But I'm glad you understand things now. And it's important that you do, because if you get this wrong, and over-code or under-code, you can get in big trouble—it might be considered fraud, and the government does not like that. Just to make things clearer, here is a table that summarizes what we just covered.

Summary of My Understanding of the E/M Coding Guidelines

Level-of-Visit Code	History	Exam	Medical Decision-Making	Medicare Payment to Physician (in Maryland)	Effect on Doctor
99212	HPI: 1–3 ROS: NA PFSH: NA	1–5 elements, system of complaint	I'm not sure	$42.80	Wife and daughter disappointed you make so little
99213	HPI: 1–3 ROS: pertinent PFSH: NA	6–11 elements, 2–4 systems	Can't figure this out, either	$75.15	The boss wants more 99214s
99214	HPI: 4+ (or 3+ chronic dz.) ROS: 2–9 PFSH: 1 element	12+ elements, 5–7 systems	Does anyone really know?	$110.66	Guilt for not listing as 99213
99215	HPI: 4+ (or 3+ chronic dz.) ROS: 10+ PFSH: 2 elements	Comprehensive, 8+ systems	Many have tried, none have succeeded	$149.03	Elation until they audit you

The Problems

Here's the very real problem with all of this. It is actually much more complicated to accurately calculate the bill for an office visit than it is to see the patient and write the SOAP note! The original challenge, if you remember, was to objectively measure the work that goes into a medical office visit. And as I stated previously, here we have an example of *a legitimate problem being addressed with a solution that is more complex than the problem itself.* In other words, the Evaluation and Management guidelines that were devised in 1995 (and revised in 1997) are far more complicated than the relatively simple SOAP note format they are based upon.

Even more important is to consider the consequences of such a complicated system. What happens when you try to use such a system in real life?

First of all, it is an unwanted and unnecessary distraction, as I have pointed out. While I am seeing a patient, a little voice pops into my head, "Did you ask enough questions to get the 99213?" or "Maybe if you ask a couple of more questions, or examine another body part, you can get the 99214." I can guarantee you that that is what is going through your doctor's head. It is just human nature.

Remember my initial training session dealing with all of this? Well, shortly thereafter I actually had to start seeing patients, and then had to calculate the level-of-visit code and fill out my own superbills. What did I do? I tried to use the coding algorithm as best I could, but it was just too complicated. I couldn't do it, especially not for the three to four patients I eventually saw per hour. So, I did what I think most doctors end up doing. I guessed! If it seemed like a pretty basic appointment, I used a 99213. If the appointment seemed complicated enough, I used a 99214. Then, I would go back and make sure that my documentation matched the level that I guessed the level of visit should be. Over the years, I picked up some tips and tricks that made my guessing more accurate. But still, it was essentially guessing.

Another thing I did was that, if there was any question in my mind about the level of the visit, I tended to down-code it to the lower level. Most doctors I have spoken to over the years end up doing the same thing. You see, most doctors do not want to cheat (there are exceptions, of course, as discussed below). But, if we have to make a choice, most of us choose to undercharge rather than risk overcharging. So, if we question whether a visit is a 99213 or a 99214, we are much more likely to use the 99213. In fact, both over-coding and under-coding are a violation of the law for which you can be prosecuted (like I will be after federal officials read this).

Also, we all hear stories about doctors who get audited (and sharply penalized) because they used too many 99214 level codes, or even 99215s. Our coding is supposed to follow a bell-shaped curve with 99213 visits at the top of the curve. In an effort to comply with this expectation, I think most of us throw in a lot of extra 99213s.

What this ultimately means is that CMS's original goal of obtaining more accurate data about the work that physicians perform during an office visit goes unmet. Because the system is too complicated to use, the data is inherently inaccurate. And there is no point to collecting data that is inaccurate.

As time went along, I did refine my knowledge regarding the E/M coding guidelines, but I would never say that my coding was more than educated guessing combined with tricks that I picked up from other physicians and from practice management journals. I just couldn't digest all of the rules, but more important, it was just not realistic to think that we could use such an overly complicated system in the throes of patient care, which was complicated enough on its own.

Another natural but unfortunate and unintended consequence of having such a complicated system for medical billing was the birth, and then the exponential growth, of the medical billing industry. Administering such a complicated system ultimately requires that physicians' practices hire medical-coding and billing staff. Almost all medical organizations were forced to hire and train huge billing departments. In addition, every payer in the medical system—the insurance companies, Medicare, and Medicaid—need such staff on their ends, as well. So having such complicated billing regulations created the need for an entirely new industry to administer the system, increasing the costs of medical care substantially!

The system also promotes fraud. Unscrupulous physicians (the exceptions mentioned previously), capitalizing on the complexity of the level-of-visit coding requirements, inappropriately up-code for more costly services than are actually provided. In 2012, the Center for Public Integrity released the results of a study that estimated that Medicare had paid over $11 billion in inflated charges related to up-coding over the previous ten years. CMS and the commercial insurances have dramatically increased their policing efforts and their expenditures to catch and prosecute this and other types of fraudulent billing practices in response. In 2015, the government's Health Care Fraud and Abuse Control Program convicted 613 defendants and collected over $1.9 billion in fraud settlements and judgments. The program received $279.7 million in mandatory funding and $672 million in discretionary funding that year.

But what the government contends is up-coding may just have been physicians finally learning how to use the coding system properly, aided by computers. Many physicians today, myself included, use EHR systems that automate the level-of-visit calculation. In 2009, when I began to use my current EHR system, I recognized almost immediately that my previous approach had likely resulted in under-coding. In fact, we had probably been substantially underpaid prior to using a computerized system (but no one at CMS had seemed to mind that). What is assumed to be fraudulent billing today may just be a reflection of physicians finally having an accurate coding tool. But many physicians today, even those using computerized medical-record systems, still hand calculate the level-of-visit code and still fill out a paper superbill.

I remember making a presentation to a group of physicians about my own company's EHR system, which by 2010 we were beginning to market. One of the chief selling points of the system was more accurate (i.e., higher) E/M coding. We did a brief analysis of these doctors' pre-EHR coding habits and found that, in their confusion about coding, and in the fear that they would be audited if they over-coded, they were grossly under-coding, using the 99212 code for most visits. They were being terribly underpaid for the work that they were doing, and they were struggling financially as a direct result. We were able to show them that they would increase their revenues by an incredible amount just by coding more accurately. Still, most of these physicians were so intimidated by the thought of using a computer, as well as of other new bureaucratic requirements affecting physicians, that the majority of them decided to retire instead! They were not alone, unfortunately. Many physicians are making the same decision because of growing administrative burdens, and that is both a shame and an issue of national significance in the setting of physician shortages.

The unintentional consequences of the system do not end there. Doctors working for large health systems are pressed by their administrators in at least two different ways as a result of the complexities of the visit coding system. In the first place, they are pushed to code at the highest levels possible. In fact, many doctors are paid using a relative value unit (RVU) calculation that takes how much they bill for their patient care into account, resulting in constant pressure to code at the highest possible levels. In addition, large health-care organizations have their own internal auditors to ensure that physicians include enough documentation in their notes to justify how much they are billing. To assist the auditors, physicians are pushed to include as much information as possible in their SOAP note documentation, both to comply with E/M coding requirements (and avoid charges of fraud), and also to make the auditors' jobs less difficult! As a result, doctors' notes are growing in length and now include all manner of information that has nothing to do with the medical care of the patient. What an incredible distraction and a waste of time, effort, and focus!

So, we see that an overly complicated level-of-visit coding system not only distracts doctors, but also results in inaccurate data, and increases costs to the medical system by necessitating two new industries, the medical billing industry and the anti-fraud industry. These are the natural consequences of such a poorly designed system.

The Fix

So in summary, the E/M Documentation Guidelines, mandated by CMS and one of the foundations of our medical payment system, are so complicated that they defeat their own purpose. They torpedo their own ship. The original intent of the system has been lost. In other words, it is a bad system that must be fixed.

Fixing this unfortunate system used to be a topic of almost constant discussion among medical professionals. But things have gotten so much worse in so many other areas of health-care administration, and physicians have been so beaten down, I think, that this aspect of the system receives little of the attention it once did. Fixing how we get paid, however, remains one of the keys to improving the American health-care system. If getting paid were simpler, physicians and their staff could focus more on patient care. And a simplified, more accurate system could save billions of health-care dollars to the nation.

So, let's take the opportunity to imagine how we might make things right. Since this is the first time we are dealing with *the fix* in this book, we should take some time to discuss the general approach we should take. Every time I begin an important project, I find that it helps to have a mission. What are our goals? What would we hope to achieve in an improved system? This is incredibly important to establish at the outset. There need to be principles that guide us toward improved health care.

I think that any fix should support and be measured against three overriding goals:

1. Increased access to care
2. Lower cost of care
3. Improved quality of care

In addition, any fix should strive to simplify our complicated, disjointed health-care system. In health care, complexity kills; simplicity saves lives. Certainly, one of the goals of an improved health-care administrative system should be to remove the distractions away from health care itself.

And simplifying this system would be easy! We should reduce the five-tiered level-of-visit coding scheme (i.e., 99211–99215), discussed above in such painful detail, from five codes to two, or three at the most. There would be a simple office visit and a complicated office visit, mirroring the way most physicians think about medical appointments anyway. The definition of each would be straightforward. A simple office visit code would be used to designate an appointment with one or two complaints (like a cough and a knee injury) or one or two simple chronic diagnoses, like high blood pressure and high cholesterol, where those complaints were relatively straightforward. The complicated office visit code would be used for an appointment with more than two straightforward complaints (or more than two chronic diagnoses), or for a more complicated complaint that requires a more thorough history and exam, such as a headache, dizziness, or abdominal pain. And any combination of three or more complaints would be considered a complicated visit. Doctors would still be required to document their care using the SOAP note format, but they would not be required, nor would they feel the need, to make their notes longer than necessary in order to satisfy a complicated coding scheme, or their auditors for that matter.

You could learn this system in just a few minutes. There would be a profound decrease in the need for training, both for medical professionals and for the billing industry (if that would still be needed). And because the system is so simple, it would be more difficult to defraud.

And, if you priced this simple system appropriately, there would be much less incentive to commit fraud. Currently, a level 99213 appointment for a Medicare patient pays a little over $75 and a 99214 pays about $110. Because that differential is so great, physicians always want the higher visit. There is a clear enticement to up-code.

If that differential in pricing were smaller, there would be less impetus to fudge the code. Let's say that, in the current system, doctors code two-thirds of visits as 99213 and one-third as 99214; then the average pay is about $95. If, in the new simpler system, we paid $90 for the simple visit and $100 for the complicated visit, this much smaller differential in pay would greatly diminish any incentive to fudge the data. It would also diminish the effect of any abuses.

So, we have the level-of-visit-coding fiasco solved. We took five codes down to two and simplified things in a profound way. Next, let's take a crack at all those code sets (new patient codes, established patient codes, sets of codes for each place of service, preventive service codes, etc.).

It turns out that all of these code sets are a vestige of a paper-based world—the time before computers (or at least good computers). If we just let computers do what they can now do, we can eliminate almost all of these extra code sets. The current system required multiple code sets, and multiple codes within each code set, because it was a paper-based system. In a paper system, there is no easy way to distinguish types of visits by things like age or place of service, except to have a unique code for each one.

So, we have separate code sets for new and established patients, and for each place of service (the doctor's office, home visits, etc.). But with a computerized system, there is no need for this. A computer can easily distinguish between a patient's first visit and subsequent visits, so there is no need for separate codes for new and established patients. Similarly, a simple check box could be used to indicate the place of service (if it was outside the office; the office would be the typical default for most physician visits). So, there is no reason that we can't reduce the separate code sets for new and established patients, and the different places of service, down to just one set of codes.

Preventive care visits, such as children's well-child checks and adult wellness exams, have their own completely separate set of codes. There are currently two sets of preventive visit codes, one for new patients and one for established patients, and then each of these code sets has seven different individual codes, stratified by age. Once again, with modern computers there is no need for all of these separate codes. A computer can easily distinguish new and established patients (as above), as well as the age of the patient. So, it is not necessary to have more than one code to denote a preventive care visit.

So, with that, we have reduced an incredibly cumbersome, difficult to comprehend system, rife with opportunities for errors and fraud, into a simple, entirely more functional one. This entire fixed system would boil down to two level-of-visit codes (simple, complicated) and one preventive visit code. You can immediately understand the entire system and could even explain it to someone else. That is elegance, and that would revolutionize medical billing and payment.

Does it satisfy the goals of our improved system? I would argue that it would go a long way toward doing just that. It is clearly a simplified approach, and would be far less of a distraction. Administering such a system would be far less expensive, which is key. If we spent less time and money administering our dysfunctional system, we could take care of more patients, increasing access to care, and be able to spend more time on improving the quality of care.

See? We can do this.

CHAPTER 3

Getting Paid—Part 2: The Worst, Most Wasteful, Guaranteed-to-Fail, You-Can't-Be-Serious Medical Billing System

I n "Getting Paid—Part 1," we learned about the distracting and destructive nature of the bizarrely complicated system used to calculate how much a doctor can charge for an appointment. Well, in terms of actually getting paid, that was just the tip of the iceberg. In "Getting Paid—Part 2," we examine the rest of the worst, most wasteful, guaranteed-to-fail, you-can't-be-serious American medical billing system.

Credentialing Kills

Before any commercial health insurance, Medicare, or Medicaid will pay a doctor or any other health-care professional new to a practice, each must first give its approval via an official credentialing process.

To become credentialed, a doctor must typically fill out an application, submit one's medical school diploma and a copy of an up-to-date state medical license, and show proof of malpractice insurance, among other things. It just so happens that there is a national database of all of this information that is maintained by an organization called the Coalition for Affordable Quality Healthcare (CAQH) as part of an effort to make credentialing across the nation more uniform and efficient. Despite that, it is neither. The word used most often to describe credentialing is "nightmarish."

Credentialing of each clinician is also required for any new practice, so when we opened our small practice in 2009, we got a bird's-eye view of the process. "Nightmarish" indeed turned out to be an accurate descriptor. We had been warned ahead of time that it was a long and arduous task, that we best start early, and that we were advised to have professional help if possible. Delays and errors are common. We were told that the process usually took ninety days, but to be careful, we should give it longer. Ninety days or longer seems like an awfully long time for such things in this day and age, doesn't it?

Our office was slated to open in July, and we began the credentialing process with commercial insurers in November (that's eight months before—I didn't want to take any chances). There were separate applications for each insurance company, each with its own nuances and potential pitfalls. Initially, we applied to twelve different commercial insurances. Medicare is an entirely different beast—you are not allowed to begin credentialing with Medicare until thirty days prior to your start date. Oddly, they are upfront about the fact that they typically take at least sixty days to complete their process. How nice that they have a process that guarantees that you won't be paid for your services for at least thirty days. Who doesn't mind not being paid for a month? Wouldn't it make sense, if the process takes sixty days, to allow us to begin sixty days prior to opening? I'm sure they have their reasons, though (like they enjoy screwing us).

The fact that you will not get paid until you are credentialed means this is all a very real problem. Being credentialed is kind of crucial if you want to be able to pay for things like rent and supplies or if you want to pay your staff, or even yourself. It makes bringing in new clinicians to a practice exceptionally challenging. It suffices to say that this aspect of getting my practice up and running made me nervous. I was nervous about lots of things at that time, but getting paid caused the most anxiety because everyone complained that it was such a difficult process.

Heeding the advice we were given, we hired a professional to manage the process for us. We gathered all of the necessary documents, filled out the necessary forms, and waited. Periodically, we got together with our pro, who reviewed a detailed spreadsheet that showed where things stood with each of the insurers. We comforted ourselves with the knowledge that I had already been credentialed with literally every one of the insurers in my previous practices (which ultimately made no difference). And, except that I was opening a new practice, nothing else had changed about me. All of the documentation we provided had been seen before by each of the companies, and the same information was available, as I said, on this CAQH website, to which each of the insurers had access. It should have been easy, right?

With a little over a month to go before we opened our doors, we were not yet credentialed with any of the insurance companies! Remember I said that I was anxious about things? This made me really, really anxious. I think I set an anxiety record of some sort. At about that time, one of the insurers happened to notice that they never received our application. That was upsetting. We had checked previously, and had been assured that everything was okay—it clearly wasn't. We resubmitted everything. I kind of wondered why this wasn't brought to our attention sooner, but what's the use of questioning things like this? It's so common that it's like a tradition of sorts. All too slowly, we began to hear from the insurers, and my credentialing crept forward. With literally just days to spare, most of the insurers began to notify us of our successful credentialing. With some effort, we were also able to get assurances from most of the insurers that we would be paid retroactively for any delays or problems that cropped up at that point. Still, it was an incredibly harrowing experience. We had booked as many patient appointments in advance as we could, but we didn't really know if we would be paid for many of them.

Let's talk about Medicare. Medicare is the government insurance for seniors that is generally highly thought of and renowned for its efficiency and low overhead. Medicare was of particular importance because my beloved senior patients make up the largest percentage of my practice, by a long shot. As I said, we were not even allowed to submit our credentialing application to Medicare until thirty days prior to our opening even though the process takes an average of sixty days. I can assure you we submitted our application on the first day we were allowed. I hounded my poor wife, our practice manager, about every thirty seconds to make sure it was done. She did not appreciate this.

Our office opened on July 9, 2009, so we should have been credentialed by Medicare on August 9, which was the thirty-fifth anniversary of Richard Nixon's resignation, by the way. That was all we got to celebrate that day because we were not yet credentialed by Medicare. Not to worry, though. I had anticipated disasters like this in my business plan. We had saved, borrowed, and begged to accumulate start-up money. And to save on expenses, I was not taking a salary during those early days. My wife and I had enough money to get by until early winter. So, why would I be worried on August 9?

Because by September 9, and then October 9, I was still not credentialed, that's why. It's okay, though, we received our first Medicare payments on November 1. They owed us a lot of money by then (they paid us retroactively for every patient we had seen, thankfully), and finally it began to come in. I would say that the process left a bit of a bitter taste in my mouth, though. Fortunately, things went pretty well for our practice after that—for a while.

In 2013, though, we decided to part ways with my original partner, which entailed, from a legal standpoint, starting over with a new practice name and tax ID. Unfortunately, that meant recredentialing all over again. Again, we started the process early. Again, we provided every insurer with all of those same documents. Our original credentialing specialist was unavailable, but we were able to find another, who assured us she knew what she was doing. We were slated to start the new practice on January 1, 2014. Unfortunately, in September my wife received a package from an insurer detailing that our "pro" had not provided most of the required information. At that point, in fact, we stopped hearing from our credentialing specialist. In a panic, and at this late date, my wife took over the process.

Once again, Medicare proved to be our biggest problem. We actually tried to submit our application to them a couple of days early. The one thing they turned out to be very efficient at doing, however, was catching an early application. It was sent back to us, and we had to resubmit the entire thing on December 1.

By the middle of January, we had not heard anything back from Medicare about our application. I found this disconcerting. We had not been paid since January 1, which, again, makes it challenging to run your business. But we also knew the process generally took sixty days. I decided to bug them. I'm glad I did. I was informed that there had been an issue with our application. Why we only found out about this when I called I'm not sure. Oh yes, because Medicare stinks at credentialing!

Only with great effort were we able to uncover the problem—that we may have submitted the wrong form—an 855I instead of the 855R (horrors). It was slightly more interesting than that, however.

Our credentialing was definitely being held up because someone determined that we used the incorrect form, yet no one at Medicare that we spoke to could definitively tell us which of these forms was correct. By mid-February, our pay having been held up for six weeks, and as yet no answer, we were in a state of near panic over our bureaucratic hell. Finally, after speaking to numerous Medicare staff who were not sure of the answer to this all-important 855I/855R question, a wise-sounding gentleman came to the phone. He had the voice and reassuring manner of Morgan Freeman when he plays God. He assured me that the 855I was the proper form. Thank God (and Morgan Freeman), we thought. We just needed to check back early the next week, and the issue should be fixed. Except that the next week I spoke to a different person who flip-flopped back to the 855R! I am not making this up. Apparently, even God doesn't know which is the correct form.

We did not get paid by Medicare until April 1, which seemed somehow appropriate (April Fools' Day). By that point, I was so bitter that I liked to say to each person at Medicare that I spoke to, "How would it be for you if we didn't pay you for four months?"

Setting Our Prices—I Can't Tell You about That

Anyway, that's enough about that pesky credentialing. Let's move on to another topic that you might think would be simple—setting a medical practice's prices. It's kind of an interesting topic.

First of all, insurance companies determine the maximum they will pay for a doctor's services, so in that sense, a medical practice's prices don't really matter. What matters is that an insurance company pays the lesser of the amount for which they are billed or the maximum they are willing to pay. If you send them a bill for less than they typically pay, they will only pay this lesser amount. So, when a doctor sets her prices, she has to choose a number that is greater than any insurance company would pay for that service. Oh, and a practice is only allowed to have one set of prices. A doctor can't charge a different amount for each insurance company (even though each insurance company pays whatever it wants), or for people who don't have insurance. So, people who can't afford insurance are doubly penalized—the ones who can afford it the least have to pay full price, and that price is higher than anyone else ends up paying!

But what really makes things tricky for the doctor is that it's difficult, and sometimes even impossible, to find out how much an insurance company intends to pay. And on top of that, a doctor is prohibited from asking other practices either how much they charge or how much they are being paid by an insurance company. I was told that speaking to any other doctor about such things is considered collusion, and it is illegal. I find this concept of collusion to be rather comical, though. An insurance company has information on literally millions of customers, knows what every practice and every doctor charges, and is thousands of times larger than a small practice like mine. But, if I speak to another doctor to find out how much they charge their patients, I have broken the law by colluding with them.

I found this out when I naïvely called a local practice manager to see how much I should charge. She began to whisper, "I can't talk to you about that." I also contacted a number of my insurers and asked them how much they paid. They acted as if this were some sort of mystery. Some of them said they didn't know, but they could look into it (it was like I was the first person who ever asked the question). Some of them outright told me that they couldn't tell me. One of them told me that their price list had been sent as an appendix to my contract. I looked at this appendix and it was blank.

So, without knowing what was reasonable to charge, and knowing that I had to come up with amounts that were higher than any insurance company might pay, I decided that my only choice was a set of prices that were extraordinarily high. It's what all medical facilities do. This is one of the reasons that there is such a discrepancy on your insurance explanation of benefits (EOB) form (if you've ever looked at it) between the amount the medical facility bills and what the insurance company pays. The problem with such a system, besides that it's just stupid, is that, as I previously stated, I also have to charge that inordinately high price to uninsured patients, who can afford it the least!

Not quite what I'd call the free market at work.

You're Not Going to Believe This, but This Is How We Get Paid (or Not)

Next, we need to talk about the overly complicated, soul-crushing process a doctor goes through in order to get paid for a medical appointment. Once you understand the details of how a doctor gets paid, the problems with the system become self-evident. But so too do the possible solutions.

Once again, I think it is very important to put this process into proper perspective. We go through the following multistep, error-prone process in an effort to collect, on average, about $75 per appointment. I am not complaining about that amount, but I certainly complain that we have to work this hard to collect such a small amount of money. And most doctors see somewhere between twenty and thirty patients in a day, so the overall amount of work that goes into getting paid is considerable.

The basic process is outlined below. Each step has its own nuances and pitfalls that can and do result in denied claims and lost billings. To make matters worse, it is well known that insurance companies (and Medicare) deny claims in error a significant percentage of the time, and each one of these steps offers an opportunity to do that. Such a complicated system is destined to fail frequently, and it fulfills its destiny. If I were a more cynical person, I might suspect that it was set up to do just that (both Medicare and insurance companies save money when denied claims don't get paid). I try not to be that cynical, but it gets harder all the time. I think you'll see what I'm talking about. Here are the bare-bones steps we go through in order to get our $75:

1. Check eligibility
2. Collect co-pay
3. Create claim
4. Receive payment (or denial) from primary insurance
5. Receive payment (or denial) from secondary insurance
6. Fight denials

From a billing perspective, we have two overriding goals with each patient we see. Number one is to collect as much as is feasible at the time of the appointment (usually in the form of co-pays and balances due). Any amount that we don't collect at that time we have to bill for, and billing takes extra time and costs money. And sometimes we don't receive payment, or it takes a lot of work to get it.

The second goal is to avoid denied claims. A denied claim is bad because it can take a lot of work to reverse the denial, and in some instances that doesn't happen. Medical practices lose a substantial amount of the money they are owed because of this. That's right, we do the work, but we don't get paid, and it's always because of some stupid technicality. Yes, that pisses me off.

Checking Eligibility

So in the two days prior to an appointment, we check every patient's insurance to make sure they do, in fact, have insurance, that the policy is up to date, and that they can come to our practice. We have to do this because at least a few times each week someone will show up who has a lapsed policy or inaccurate policy information, such as listing the wrong primary care provider, and we won't get paid. We maintain a spreadsheet of about seventy insurers and the login information to get on their websites. Most of the insurers' websites are easy to navigate, but some can make it very difficult to obtain this basic information that we need.

Even after verifying that a patient is eligible as best we can, they may turn out not to be! More than once, we have been listed "in network" on an insurance website, and in fact, we were not. Those claims are denied even though it is the fault of the insurance company. We have also been listed as "out of network" when we were clearly in the network. What should be a simple matter can become an incredible hassle.

For our two-provider practice, checking eligibility takes approximately an hour and a half per day. That is a lot of time to have to spend just to see if patients are properly insured.

Collecting Co-Pays

When patients come to their appointments, we check them in, and we make every attempt to collect the co-pay, which is usually an amount between $10 and $40. Unfortunately, at least a few times per day, a patient doesn't bring any money, or even a credit card, and they have to be billed. A certain percentage of these patients never pay, of course.

Think about this. Would you go to the store, or the gas station, without money? So why is it that people regularly go to a doctor's office without it? Of course, some people just don't have the money. But also, I think that health care is an odd "business," in that it's not just a business, but a business that has to do with people's health. Because of that, I think that patients intuitively know that we behave differently (i.e., we look past the fact that you didn't bring any money and take care of you anyway).

There can also be co-pay confusion. For instance, our practice's two most popular commercial insurers each now have a wellness plan, and patients who participate don't have a co-pay (the insurer pays it). But we have no reliable way of knowing which patients are participants—we are not usually notified in any way—and some patients are unclear about it, as well. What ends up happening, therefore, is that some patients pay a co-pay who didn't have to, and some don't pay who should have. Fun!

My Happy Place . . . Getting Paid

Once the patient has paid their co-pay (or not), they get to see me. From a billing perspective, at least two things must come from every medical visit: the level-of-visit code, about which you learned more than you ever wanted to know in the previous chapter, and the diagnosis code (or codes), about which you will learn more than you ever wanted to know in a little while. The level-of-visit code and the diagnosis code(s) are the minimum information necessary to create a claim, the term we use for a medical bill. For your sake, I'm going to grossly oversimplify things and just say that a claim is created and gets sent to the insurance company for payment.

Let's start with the happier subject—getting paid. This does happen most of the time, thankfully, though it's often a lot more complicated than you would think. Part of that complication is that Medicare and the commercial insurances each do things their own way, and Medicare is administered in different regions by different commercial insurers, and each of them does things slightly differently, so that needs to be considered as well. In other words, there are different sets of rules for each insurer, and there are lots of insurers. In our small practice, we accept close to forty!

Let's discuss getting paid by Medicare first. I think you'll agree that this is an awfully complicated process to go through for $75. To emphasize the point, I want you to try to hold your breath while you read this next paragraph. Traditional Medicare pays only 80 percent of a claim (so let's say you receive $60 of the total $75 in this first round). The remaining 20 percent ($15) is either paid by the patient (hopefully at the time of the appointment; otherwise, it gets billed) or a bill gets sent to a secondary insurance company. Just to make things interesting here, some of the secondary insurances also include a small co-pay amount, which, like other co-pays, we try to collect at the time of the visit. The remaining claim amount ($10–$15) "crosses over" to the secondary insurance automatically (electronically) about 80 percent of the time, depending on the insurer. The remaining 20 percent do not cross over automatically. For these, we need to print out a secondary claim form, which we combine with the primary insurer's explanation of benefits (EOB), which then gets sent to the secondary insurance either electronically or by mail. That was complicated, right? Take a few breaths now.

Getting paid by a commercial insurance company is different. About 70 percent of the time we are paid the full balance, and nothing else has to happen (hurray). But about 30 percent of the time, there is either a missed co-pay or the patient owes a deductible amount. Most of the time, this amount is billed directly to the patient, but sometimes a patient has a secondary insurance that we have to bill instead. Most of the time the secondary insurance pays the full amount owed, but a small percentage of the time there is yet another remaining balance due, and this gets billed to the patient directly (this is often an amount of about $10-$12).

Even when we get our hands on the money, though, it's not all fun and games. Then we have to apply the payments. You see, we have an accounts receivable entry in our billing system for every patient visit (on an average day that is about thirty-five visits in our two-provider practice). Each one of those entries needs to be closed out. When we receive a payment from Medicare or an insurance company, it might be for just one visit or it may cover multiple patients and appointments. We have to go through each check, and divide up the amounts among the accounts receivable entries. This isn't hard to do, but it is time-consuming, taking three to four hours per day, which is a lot of time!

Believe it or not, that was a simplified version of getting paid. All that work for $75! It feels like we put in about $500 worth of work to collect it. And, if a claim gets denied, sometimes we actually do put in $500 worth of work to get $75 (if we can successfully fight the denial)!

Don't Go into Denial

A denied claim is often just pure getting-paid hell. But in medical billing, denials are a way of life. In a system that is so complicated, it is just hard to know all of the rules that affect billing and payment, and it is harder still to know each insurer's idiosyncratic interpretation of these rules. Naturally, there are a great many opportunities for disagreements and errors, along with arbitrary and inconsistent application of the rules.

But I also think that insurance companies capitalize on the complexity, even using it to their advantage in a managerial technique I refer to as "systematic incompetence." Knowing that the system is so complicated and prone to error, insurers could spend time and money trying to improve the system or devise better training, so that billing and coding rules would be enforced in a more consistent manner and so that errors could be kept to a minimum. Or they could take the opposite approach and merely turn a blind eye to the dysfunction. They might believe that it is to their advantage to allow the incompetence to continue. It is certainly true that the more denied claims there are, and the harder it is to fix a denied claim, the less the insurer ends up paying to doctors, and the more profit they make. Based on what I've seen, I believe the latter situation is likely. In other words, I believe that "systematic incompetence" is for real.

If you spent any time attempting to adjudicate denied claims (my wife does this much of the day for our practice), you might agree. When we first received notice that some of our claims were being denied, we contacted the insurance company billing department to try to settle the issue. We were told that we used incorrect billing codes. When we asked what the correct codes were, the reply was "We're not allowed to tell you." Other times that we received a denial, we contacted the billing department, received an explanation of the problem, and resubmitted the claim, only to have it denied once more. We called again, but this time, received an entirely different explanation.

Denials are a huge problem nationwide that creates an incredible amount of waste and unnecessary expense. Medicare has a claim denial rate of close to 5 percent. Most commercial insurers have lower denial rates than that, but still, with the huge number of medical appointments that occur every day in this country, even a low rate can have a huge impact. And a significant proportion of those denials represent errors made by insurance companies. The American Medical Association in 2013 estimated that between 2010 and 2013, "$43 billion dollars could have been saved if commercial insurers consistently paid claims correctly."

There are lots of reasons that claims get denied: unapproved services, insurance ineligibility, incorrect spelling of patient names, incorrect birth dates, provider out of area, unapproved diagnostic codes, incorrectly entered codes, and incorrect code modifiers, to name just a few.

There's No Denying They Are Good at Denials

Remember I said previously that you would learn more than you ever wanted to know about diagnostic codes? Now is that time. Incorrect diagnosis codes are one of the most common reasons claims are denied. You see, every medical diagnosis has a corresponding code (or in some cases multiple codes) in the International Classification of Disease code set (we are on the tenth edition, so the common abbreviation is ICD-10). To get paid, you must submit at least one of these diagnostic codes for each service you provide. So, a diagnosis of sore throat becomes code J02.9. High blood pressure is coded I10. That seems easy enough, right? But an ankle sprain has to be coded for the side of the body (S93.402 for left and S93.401 for right) and is broken down into a first-visit code (left ankle sprain, first visit, is S93.402A), a subsequent-visit code S93.402D (why isn't the second visit a "B"?), and sequelae from a left-ankle sprain are coded S93.402S.

The diagnostic codes can and do get complicated from a billing perspective. First of all, there are sixty-eight thousand ICD-10 codes to choose from. That's a lot. With that many codes, sometimes it is just flat-out hard to find the right code. With the advent of computerized medical records, finding most diagnostic codes today is usually relatively easy. But there are some exceptions. Ironically, I have a hell of a time finding the correct codes for almost any fracture (there are so many codes to describe every fracture that it's nearly impossible to find the right one), but I have no problem pulling up the codes for such uncommon—I hope—diagnoses as "struck by a golf club," code W21.13XA; "erotic vomiting" (whatever that is; I don't judge), which is code F65.89; and my personal favorite, "hit by object falling from aircraft, without accident to aircraft, occupant of spacecraft injured," code T14.90.

But it is very important to use the "correct" code, because some of the codes are not considered billable (so why do we have them?), or one insurance company may accept a particular code, while another does not, and that distinction is usually completely arbitrary. Choose the wrong code for the wrong insurance, and you get a rejected claim, which as I noted, is bad.

At various times, we have had the code for obesity (code E66.9) rejected (most insurances don't pay for treatment of obesity, believe it or not); for many insurances, tobacco use (code F17.200) is not a valid code because smoking cessation is often not covered. That's correct, people, treating the two most significant risk factors—obesity and tobacco use—for the number one killer in America—heart disease—is often not covered! We have also had mental-health codes rejected, either because the service is not covered or because the patient is required to see a psychiatrist, despite the fact that there may be no psychiatry appointments available for months at a time.

Another reason that diagnostic codes result in denied claims is that they lack the necessary "specificity." One of the reasons the US moved from the ICD-9 code set to ICD-10 was the perceived need for more specific information about the types of conditions that are being treated by American doctors. And one of the reasons that we went from thirteen thousand codes in the ICD-9 system to sixty-eight thousand codes is that in the ICD-10 code set many general diagnoses are broken down into multiple, more specific, subcodes. So congestive heart failure (CHF) can be coded I50.9 for nonspecific CHF, but is also broken down into a multitude of sub-diagnoses, like I50.31 for acute diastolic CHF or I50.1 for acute left-sided CHF. Insurance companies will deny a claim if they feel the diagnosis is not specific enough. But, in the example above regarding CHF, we often don't know which subtype we are dealing with (even most cardiology notes that I read don't list the diagnosis to this level of specificity); despite that, if we don't use the "correct" code, we run the risk of a rejected claim. This represents somewhat of a quandary, of course.

One other diagnostic-code nuance that I will mention (there are a lot of them) is that some diagnoses must be paired with others in order to qualify for payment. For instance, when patients see me for a tick bite—I practice in Lyme disease country, so this is a frequent occurrence—to be paid, I have to list the code for the bite, which has unique codes for different locations of the body, but also have to include a code for the "place of occurrence," meaning where the person was when they were bit (Y92.821 indicates the forest as the place of occurrence). The following conversation takes place far too often as a consequence.

Me: "Where were you bit?"

Patient: "On my leg."

Me: "I mean where were you when you were bit?"

Patient: "I don't know. I'm outside a lot."

Me: "I have to know so that I can bill your visit."

Patient: "I'm not sure. Do you want me to make it up?"

One insurance company requires that we include onset dates for certain types of diagnoses. No other company requires onset dates. It is very easy, therefore, to make mistakes with this company's claims, and we do, from time to time.

Medicare has made it essentially impossible for me to get paid for procedures that I perform in my office. They deny the claims, and the reason given is that we haven't included the name of a referring physician. We didn't include that information because no one referred the patients to me. I am a primary care doctor, and my patients just show up on their own. When we contacted Medicare to discuss this, we were told that we should list me as the referring physician. That doesn't make sense, of course, but we've learned not to let things like not making sense bother us anymore. So, we listed my name as the referring physician's. The claims still got denied! We have never been able to receive a straight answer about this, so I don't bill Medicare anymore for procedures!

Medicare has also made it nearly impossible for us to get paid for giving tetanus shots. As a primary care clinician, I was taught to monitor and maintain every patient's immunizations. But we find that insurances, especially Medicare, can make the process so mysterious (and we spend thousands of dollars to purchase immunizations, so we can lose a substantial amount of money if we are not paid), and we have had so many claims for tetanus shots denied, that we are hesitant to provide this extremely important service. I have never seen a case of tetanus, by the way, but I hear that it's pretty vicious—and uniformly deadly. One of the classic signs of tetanus is *risus sardonicus*, which Wikipedia describes as "the appearance of raised eyebrows and an open 'grin'—which can appear sardonic or malevolent to the lay observer—displayed by those suffering from these muscle spasms." If Medicare continues to make it so hard for people to get their tetanus shots, maybe I will see this someday (which would be a tragedy, of course).

Based on our experiences with denied claims, we have developed an interesting, though counterintuitive, workaround to medical billing—we don't bill for a number of the services that we provide. As I have said, the worst thing that can happen is a denial, because any one denial can result in hours of fruitless work, huge frustration, and still, we might not get paid. Over the years, we have found that the fancier we try to be with a claim, and the more services we attempt to capture, the more likely it is that a claim will be denied. Therefore, we often skip billing for certain services (like certain procedures or office-based testing), and just bill the simple office visit, which is unlikely to get denied (even though we performed a procedure as well as the simple office visit). How's that for a business philosophy? But it's the type of choice you end up making in this nonsense system. We lose some money this way—we're not getting paid for some of the work that we do—but it is better to lose a little (the procedures) than a lot (the whole visit). And we are more likely to retain what is left of our sanity.

Don't Worry, It Gets Worse

I have to give them credit because the evil geniuses at the insurance companies really do think of everything. Besides denying claims because of coding "errors," insurers, it turns out, deny claims for lots of other reasons, as well. I sometimes imagine that our brightest college graduates, no longer drawn to the sciences, are instead ending up at insurance companies, where they are using their considerable brainpower to find new and more creative ways to make the system break down. It's not just systematic incompetence anymore. It's incompetence perfected! You've got to hand it to them.

Here are some examples of what else might go wrong. Most of the problems below come from one company, one that unfortunately also happens to be one of the largest insurers in the state of Maryland. They are also the absolute worst at fixing problems when they arise. Maybe there's a connection there. Although this company is the worst of the ones we deal with, at times we face similar issues with others (or they have made up their own unique ways to deny our claims).

The number one problem we encounter stems from the fact that the company's local office serves as the administrator for claims for patients with the same company's nonlocal plans as well. And we have many patients who have these other policies, whose claims must first be processed by our local division and then subsequently "wired" (their word, not ours) to the patient's home plan. If there is any problem with the claim, the home plan then sends the claim back to our local office, which then informs us of the bad news in the form of a denial notice. We, in turn, then have to call the home plan directly, or even write a letter, asking to have the claim reconsidered. This complicated process can take months.

Unfortunately, for some reason, many issues arise with these out-of-area plans. For instance, claims from the company's West Virginia division have frequently been denied, or patients have been charged inappropriately high co-pays, when they have seen our practice's family nurse practitioner. It turned out that the West Virginia division listed her as a specialist. She is not a specialist. Multiple phone calls regarding the problem yielded no resolution. We were even told at one point that the company doesn't recognize nurse practitioners as valid providers of health care—they have since 2011! Not only do we have to deal with the insurance company when these errors occur, but we also receive complaints from patients, many of whom say that if the higher co-pays continue, they will have to switch to another practice!

At one point, my wife became so frustrated that she went on this company's Facebook page and wrote a complaint. Within a few minutes, she received an email message putting her in touch with a provider representative, who informed us that the local office had no control over the West Virginia division's claim denials. We were told that they had their own set of rules and regulations. Finally, and only with great effort, we were able to get the West Virginia division to acknowledge that they had listed our nurse practitioner as a specialist in error. Even then, it took them months to get the problem fixed, and even after all that, the errors persist from time to time.

We also have problems getting paid when this same large insurer is the secondary insurance paying on a claim. This company is one of the few insurances with which we work that doesn't accept electronic secondary claims, which means that we need to print out a paper claim and attach to the claim the primary insurance EOB, which shows how much it paid, and the balance due. This process is time-consuming in and of itself, but then the company has a tendency to lose the EOB somewhere along the way, and the claim is denied. We have mailed individual claims as many as four times, just to have them denied for the same reason. It took another post on the company's Facebook page to get a response from an analyst, who was able to get a number of the claims paid. Interesting use of social media, isn't it?

And see how you like this new one we've been noticing. Of late, some insurance companies have taken to sending patients a "Coordination of Benefits" query, in the form of a letter, which as we understand it, is to satisfy the insurer that they are, in fact, the patient's insurer and that they are correctly identified as the patient's primary or secondary payer. Payments are being held up until the patient returns the questionnaire telling the insurance company what they should already know. We don't get paid until the patient realizes that the letter, which they presume to be junk mail and therefore keep tossing in the wastebasket, isn't actually junk mail (it's debatable) and needs to be returned. Again, you've got to give them credit for being good at what they do, which, unfortunately, is ripping us off.

I'll tell you about one more remarkable way that insurance companies have figured out to keep us from getting paid. I love this one because it relies on new technology, which we tend to view favorably, and because it is actually marketed as an easier way for medical practices to receive payments, which we would also like—except that it sometimes doesn't work. The way it is supposed to work is that the insurance company, rather than sending us a musty old check, instead sends a payment card, with an appearance much like our bank and credit cards. Under separate cover, we are sent the username and password for the card, which enables us to access a special payment website. Unfortunately, sometimes the access codes haven't worked—and then we can't get paid. Then, we have to call the insurance company to report the problem, only to find that the insurance company doesn't know what the problem is! This represents a brilliant new use of technology as well as a groundbreaking new concept in nonpayment all rolled into one.

The Problem with All of This

First and foremost, I hope it is clear that this is just a stupid way to do things. Having to go through so many steps to get such relatively small amounts of money is obviously wasteful. Even for larger amounts of money, though, I don't think this is a system that makes a lot of sense. And is there any other type of business where a service is provided first and then afterwards we decide that the service was invalid and refuse payment? That's a rhetorical question, by the way. And if the answer to this rhetorical question is yes, then they should stop doing things that way.

There is just no reason in the world that it should be difficult for a doctor to get paid for her services, or even to have to bill for services at all (more on that just a little later). Enough is enough!

The most obvious drawback to such a system is the unnecessary expense it creates. Needless expenditures for medical billing are one of the most obvious reasons why health care in America is so costly, and such expenses contribute to our inability to provide care to millions of people. And people who do not have access to medical care often die as a result, so having a more functional payment system is not just sound policy, it is a moral imperative. Do we need more motivation than that?

But the effects of this system go much further. It is now tradition to tell doctors in training that "doctors are not good at business." What that really means is that doctors have had a terrible time attempting to keep up with this way of doing things. It's not that I take offense to the notion that doctors aren't good business-people, it's that the whole system is just so ridiculous. Everyone is bad at it. But more important, because of that, almost all medical practices now must have billing staff, and often cede control of their practices to professional managers, or even contract their billing out to costly billing services—all to administer a payment system that shouldn't exist. In addition, an alarming number of doctors I speak with relate horror stories regarding practice managers or billing ser-vices that have ripped them off or were just downright incompetent. So now there's that as well.

As a result, many doctors (if not most at this point) are leaving their private practices to work for large health systems as employees in the hopes that they can "just practice medicine." Most will tell you, however, that they just traded one set of problems for another. We can argue the relative merits of having doctors herded into larger groups and health systems, but this is not happening because it is a better way to deliver care (that has not been shown). It is happening as a natural consequence of this lousy system.

And worst of all, many doctors are just throwing in the towel and leaving medicine altogether, all because we have allowed an out-of-control government bureaucracy and an all-controlling insur-ance industry to run roughshod over a process that should simply be happening as an afterthought—getting paid. I guarantee that this effect of our dysfunctional medical payment system is not a desir-able outcome. But I am also confident it can be done much better.

The Fix

In fact, once you see the problems, the fix looks pretty easy, right? Throw out the current system, simplify the process, and you're pretty much done. I don't think it takes a genius to know that if we removed as many steps as possible, and whenever possible, maybe used modern technologies (that have existed for years), we could do things far better and with incredible ease.

First of all, the credentialing process that I described should not exist. There should be one single national credentialing body that maintains and administers all of a physician's information and credentials. Oh yes, that body already exists—the previously mentioned Coalition for Affordable Quality Healthcare. The fix is to use that existing service and eliminate the credentialing process by Medicare and the individual insurances entirely. If an insurance company or Medicare needed to verify a physician's credentials, the process should be limited to one or two weeks max.

The entire rest of the eligibility and medical billing process described above should, and easily could, be eliminated and replaced by a point-of-care payment and insurance photo identity card. The card could be swiped through a card reader that could both report eligibility prior to the appointment and process the payment directly following the appointment (by the way, this is already how they do it in Taiwan). In other words, eliminate the billing process entirely. And eliminate denials altogether for all usual care, including, of course, mental health services and lifestyle counseling. There should be an approved basket of care that covers all but the most extraordinary measures and cannot be denied.

If we did that, we would improve the practice of medicine profoundly, and we could reduce health-care expenditures immensely. If physician practices, both large and small, no longer had to worry and waste their valuable time and energy to deal with the basic process of getting paid, we would be capable of so much more. You might even be able to pay us less! Okay, just kidding about that.

CHAPTER 4

Computerizing Medicine— Meaningless Use

Remember I said that getting paid was all doctors ever used to gripe about? Well, getting paid may be bumped from the leaderboard by computers, more specifically, EHRs, electronic health records.

Computers were supposed to revolutionize the practice of medicine. And some day they may. But in the greatest of ironies, computers have become one of the biggest problems plaguing medical professionals. Rather than helping to fix the practice of medicine, they are one of the reasons that many physicians are leaving clinical care and even retiring early. Thanks, computers.

There are many reasons that computerization has failed so miserably. Number one is the technology itself, which most physicians would rate as essentially unusable. Magnifying that problem, though, has been government's handling of things. Early on, the problem was a shocking lack of guidance—a failure to lead where leadership was sorely needed. Then, recognizing their error, government regulators plodded in, but then wreaked havoc in a classic case of misguided overreach that will be detailed below. The extent of their failure is astonishing. The effects of their failure are incredibly far-reaching.

But before we get too far along, I should list my qualifications. For a simple country doctor, and just an average computer user, the extent of my experiences with health information technology is surprising (especially to me). It just so happens that I am one of the creators of the best electronic health record software system you've never heard of. In an odd turn of events, in 2006 I became part of a team of physicians and computer professionals who set out to create the first great EHR. Our team successfully cracked the code of EHR usability, the issue that troubles EHR users more than any other. I use the EHR in my practice, and it has taken our ability to get work done to an entirely different level, and it has improved our patients' care. I have also trained other practices and have had the opportunity to speak to many clinicians about their EHR experiences. And despite what you are about to read to the contrary, I am confident that computerized medicine will someday deliver on its great potential—once we dig out from all the damage that the federal government has done.

Paper Was Bad, but It Never Made Me Cry

The problems we associate with paper medical records are not unimportant. Good charting and documentation are the heart and soul of quality medical care, and anything that impedes this creates considerable problems. The medical chart is not just a repository of a doctor's notes—it is the all-important hub of a patient's clinical activity and communications regarding their care. The medical chart is integral to all aspects of clinical care. It contains the medical history, appointment notes, medication and allergy lists, immunization histories, test results, and hospital and specialist notes.

A well-documented, complete, and well-organized medical chart encourages good care and prevents mistakes more than any other single factor. Doctors and nurses spend a great deal of time interacting with medical charts, and therefore, any problems with them can have far-reaching effects.

The weaknesses inherent in paper medical records were obvious, as was the need for something better. Paper records, often with handwritten notes, could be illegible; were often poorly organized and incomplete; took up a great deal of space; could only be used by one person at a time; were difficult to share; and were sometimes lost. Further, extracting meaningful data from paper records was almost impossible. And managing a practice's or hospital's paper charts took a small army of people who needed to place new information and notes of all sorts into the charts; to pull the charts for appointments and messages; to transport the charts around the building(s) for various tasks; to copy them when necessary; to maintain the small city of stacked and shelved charts in the chart room; and the big task—to find wayward charts. The costs associated with all of this were substantial. But maybe worst of all, paper records could not accompany patients as they made their way to other medical facilities or on their travels.

On the other hand, I never heard a physician complain that they would be quitting the practice of medicine because their paper records were such a problem. Once the paperwork was on your desk or in your exam room, charting was usually quick and easy. Physicians did not regularly spend extra hours at night catching up charting in their paper records because they were so slow. Nor did I once hear that a paper chart had caused a physician to cry (more on that later).

It is an odd thing for me to say, but the medical chart interested me from the start. Just as an aside—when my wife and I first met, which was long before I considered going to med school, I was a singer in a band. My wife thought she was getting Mick Jagger, but what she ended up with was a medical charting maven—sigh. Anyway, my first job out of residency was as a family physician at a small-town community health clinic. I was also the organization's medical director, and therefore felt somewhat of a responsibility for our charts and what was in them, neither of which was consistently exemplary. This was the year 2000, prior to most efforts to computerize the clinical side of medicine.

The paper charts I initially encountered in that practice left something to be desired. The older ones were thick, and many of these records had fraying or torn pages, or pages that were threatening to fall out. Important information could be difficult to find and was sometimes misfiled. Older notes in those charts had been handwritten. At the time that I started practicing, the notes were being dictated into a handheld recording device and then transcribed. Transcription resulted in a typed note, which was good because it was legible. But it could take days for the typed note to return from the transcriptionist and to appear in the patient's chart. Because of this delay, we would also jot down a brief handwritten note that would go in the chart temporarily so that if the patient developed some issue prior to the arrival of the transcribed note—which was not infrequent—we would have some idea of what we had done during the recent appointment.

After each patient's appointment, I would scurry back to my office and quickly dictate my note. Other physicians might wait to dictate their notes until they had a break, or even after they were finished seeing patients. I was too worried that I would forget something to wait this long.

In 2001, I was given the opportunity to try to improve our paper charts and our approach to charting when our health center enrolled in a government-sponsored practice "re-design" collaborative. In this groundbreaking project, we were asked to examine our patients' experiences as they moved through our practice, and to see if and how we could improve things. Our initial focus was to get patients seen on a timelier basis.

We eventually turned our attention to our charts, which we set about to "re-design." Thinking about it, I realized what would become the basis of our future EHR's design—that the great majority of what we did, said, and documented in delivering medical care was patterned, repetitive, and almost entirely predictable. Most of the notes that we make in a medical chart are just slight variations of a few very similar themes. Understanding this, I created a number of forms—clinical templates that listed the most common aspects of a doctor's note as options that could be quickly checked or circled—that we then used to efficiently and effectively document each of the various types of medical appointments. This new system streamlined note creation and improved the content of the practice's charting—no small feat.

It was apparent to me that such a system of templates would lend itself very nicely to computerization. In fact, these same concepts and templates, in computerized form, would become one of the foundations of our EHR.

Our new charting system also enabled on-the-spot documentation. In other words, the new system was so convenient that we could literally chart our notes as we were seeing our patients. We no longer had to wait days to receive our transcribed notes. Nor did we require the services of transcriptionists any longer. This saved the practice about $30,000 per year. Our executive director was delighted for the sake of our bottom line. Our employees were not so delighted. They wondered, not without some merit, if further practice "improvements" might imperil their jobs.

But it was a profound and important lesson—that we could improve upon the traditional morass of paper charting, and that the impacts resonated throughout our practice.

Attack of the Computers

Having a paper charting system that was working so well for us made it possible to be selective when the first EHR systems became available and pressure began to mount to switch to an electronic system. The first such moment came in 2003, when our clinic's executive director asked me to sign off on the purchase of one such system, sight unseen. Like many EHR systems, this one was designed by a practice management (billing and scheduling) software company. Our clinic was using the company's practice management software already. The company had created a clinical EHR that interacted directly with the practice management components of their software. This notion was extremely appealing, and our executive director made a common assumption—that this idea made so much sense, and the advantages of computerization were so obvious, that all we needed to do was sign the contract and all of our dreams would come true. This same mistake was made by many around the country.

I thought much the same thing, but also thought a demonstration of the product was necessary before I could sign off on the purchase. A salesman from the company came to our office and flashed slides onto the wall displaying their EHR's clinical screens. They raved about the incredible attributes of their system. The executive director was sold.

He was disappointed when I again declined to sign off on the project, insisting that we needed to see more than a slide show—we needed to use the software in order to know if it was good or not. I asked the salesman if there was an interactive demo that I could try. The answer, surprisingly, was no. The best that they could do was to allow me to visit a practice that was already using the product. The closest such practice happened to be in Arizona. I took him up on his offer. I'm very glad that I did.

I learned two extraordinarily valuable lessons during my visit. Number one was that the EHR was essentially impossible to use. I was, at the time, a reasonably experienced computer user. The salesman set me up in front of one of their computers and gave me some pointers, but even after hours of trying, I could not make any sense of this EHR. I could not find any of the relevant clinical information that I was accustomed to viewing in a typical medical record. Nor could I figure out how I would document patient care in this system. I am glad I made that trip, because purchasing this product would have been a disaster, a very expensive disaster, for our practice.

Lesson number two was that, if we let them, computers could completely disrupt the doctor-patient relationship. During my visit, I witnessed something that I found shocking. I wanted to watch the clinical team as they used the EHR—to see the system in action. One physician agreed to let me pose as a test patient while she charted on the computer. I sat on the exam table as a patient would. The physician took her place at a desk in front of the computer, facing the wall, her back to me. She interviewed me as if I were the patient— all the time facing in the opposite direction. Not one time did the physician take her gaze from the computer. Not one time did she actually face me or make eye contact with me! I was stunned that she would allow the computer in the room to completely disrupt what I thought was an essential part of medical care—human interaction.

But the pressure to computerize was only growing. More systems were becoming available all the time. The early reports on these systems were consistent—consistently bad. The number one complaint was the considerable expense associated with purchasing a system, implementing it, and then maintaining it. Even small practices were encountering costs in the high five-digit and even low six-digit range. The effect of such large investments was that most practices and health systems that purchased an EHR then felt they had to stick with what they had, no matter the effect on clinical care or the bottom line, for the foreseeable future.

This was a shame because most EHR users found that their systems were essentially unusable. EHRs were incredibly cumbersome, often profoundly limiting the number of patients that could be seen (I heard a number of reports that physicians were only able to see half the number of patients they had previously seen even a year later). Combined with the exorbitant cost of many EHRs, the effect on practices' bottom lines was frightening. Beyond that, EHRs were so unwieldy that many physicians delayed their charting until the end of the day, spending many hours at night trying to catch up. This even spawned a new term—"pajama doctors." For many clinicians, the EHR became a nightmare that has not let up even today.

This excerpt is from a July 2015 article by Steven J. Stack, MD, president of the American Medical Association:

> Melissa Rhodes, MD, a Georgia physician in pulmonary critical care and sleep medicine, is fed up. She was an early adopter of the technology, implementing her first EHR in 2006. . . . She wanted the system to live up to its promise— but that didn't happen. . . .
>
> Dr. Rhodes tallied up how much her three-physician practice has spent on her EHR and related IT costs—over the past year, that number hit $84,000.
>
> But more important than the costs, Dr. Rhodes' EHR has limitations that affect her patients. The system won't allow her to titrate orders for patients in the intensive care unit. And she has to personally enter orders, no matter what time of day or night, without being permitted to benefit from the help of nursing colleagues at the hospital.

"There are so many orders you can't put in," she said. "It only leads to harm for patient care, and more medical errors—not less."

Understandably, against this backdrop, physicians were slow to adopt this new technology. Administrators and IT consultants criticized physicians for being resistant to change and technology-averse. We were badgered to "just get on board!" I just didn't see the point of spending an inordinate amount of money for a system that might disrupt my ability to care for my patients, could potentially rob me of any time to have a life outside of work, and hadn't been shown to improve the quality of patient care. Many other physicians apparently felt the same way.

Using the Unusable

My first experience using a commercial EHR came when I began working for a new clinic in 2008. They had been using a popular EHR for a few years already. But their experience, and then mine, mirrored what I had heard about elsewhere. Among the staff, the system generated essentially constant eye rolling and sighing.

Just getting trained to use the system was a challenge. There happened to be no training materials, which I found disturbing. The company's approach was to train one staff member as a "super user" and then allow that person to train everyone else. So, one morning I sat for a few hours with our nurse "super user," who showed me around the system. From there on out, it was up to me to learn anything else I needed to know. That afternoon it was patient appointments using the EHR.

The problem with inadequate training, in addition to making it challenging just to use the system, was that knowledge about the system was inconsistent throughout the organization. One of the system's more interesting features was that it was possible to record some of a patient's key clinical information in more than one location of the chart. And without proper training, that's exactly what people did. So, if you didn't look multiple places (or didn't know to look), you weren't sure if you had all the information you needed.

A lot of crucial patient information was also hidden from view. Past notes, certain test results, and specialist notes were stored in a vertical bar along the side of the screen. All of the information that had been entered on one date was collapsed into one line that only displayed that date, but nothing about what information, if any, lay behind the date, a click away. Only if you clicked the date did it expand to display the underlying information. But then the expanded details often took up so much space that the next date was blocked from view. To get to the next date, the original one that you had opened up had to be reduced back to the date display. It was a time-intensive task, and a confusing one. Because the information was essentially hidden from view, and because it was so challenging to access it, it was very easy to miss important data.

So, doctors and nurses went from using disorganized illegible paper records to disorganized but legible electronic charts where you might not be able to find important information. Because of poor training and a confusing design, we had lost some of the most important potential benefits of computerized charting.

But the biggest issue by far was slowness. One of the most oft-made promises by EHR salespeople (and the drooling administrators who were touting the systems—but didn't have to use them) was the increased revenue that would result from streamlined electronic charting. Well, we dreamt of the Jetsons but we got the Flintstones! Slowness was the norm. Despite that, we were expected to see our usual number of patients. This was an incredible challenge, and even became dangerous, when system-wide slowdowns were a regular occurrence. Even when the system was working, certain screens could take what seemed like forever to load.

I remember saying a silent prayer that I would not need information from certain areas of the patient's chart because the system would hang up for what felt like an eternity. All the while, the patient was sitting there, wondering why I had gone silent. I learned to avoid certain screens, but I also developed between-screen patter with the patient to reduce the awkwardness. One physician even told me that in his training he was encouraged to find other things to do, or think about things he could say, while he awaited the system's return! What was he supposed to do? Develop a hobby? Take up knitting? I wonder how much you could charge if you saw a patient for diabetes and knitted them a cardigan?

And yes, I heard a story about an experienced physician who was attempting to see a patient, but the electronic record was so slow to open, and he became so frustrated with the delay, that he began to cry. I can assure you, when you have a waiting room full of patients and your system is slow, it is maddening. I talked with a physician recently as he was opening a patient's EHR chart, and he timed how long it took—fifty-five seconds. That was about average for his system, he thought. In the days of yore, when you sat down to a paper record, it opened immediately. Now, if this physician with whom I was speaking sees twenty-five patients per day, he is spending almost an entire half hour just waiting to get into patient records! He went on to tell me that he just assumes that most days the software isn't going to work, and that way he isn't so disappointed!

"Hi, honey, what did you do today?"

"I waited."

Computer slowness has become such an accepted part of life that it has even spawned a new medical profession—the EHR scribe. The scribe follows the clinician from room to room, creating aspects of the clinical notes for them while the patient is being seen, ostensibly saving time. There are at least two problems with using a scribe, though. It is doubtful that the scribe documents the same level of detail, or the flavor of a visit, that a clinician would. But also, imagine the added expense of having to hire a scribe for each clinician because your system is so slow! So much for all that extra cash the EHR was supposed to generate.

E-prescribing was recognized as one of the most important features of computerized medicine because computer-generated prescriptions would be legible, and because the computer had the potential to prevent errors with features such as automated drug-interaction checking. Unfortunately, the e-prescribing module was the slowest and most poorly designed portion of the system I was using. I began to dread prescribing medications, which is bad because I'm a doctor! I learned to wait until the end of an appointment to write or refill any prescriptions because it was just too disruptive to sit there waiting in the middle of an appointment. Patients with long lists of medications were a nightmare. Because of the amount of time it could take, I might even skip one of the most crucial steps of any medical appointment—checking the accuracy of the patient's prescription list. That is terrible because an inaccurate medication list is one of the greatest dangers in medicine. There is no easier way to hurt a patient than to prescribe a medication without knowing what else they are taking.

Also, I found that the e-prescribing module had a very dangerous glitch—it sometimes altered the text of the instructions I had written detailing how a medication was to be taken. I am not kidding! The first few times it happened, I caught the mistake, but assumed that it was my own error. I soon learned that it was, indeed, a computer glitch. It occurred only with certain medications. I tried to be diligent to always catch the error. Unfortunately, one time I did not. A patient called a couple of weeks after I had started her on an antidepressant, Effexor XR, saying that she did not feel well since starting the medication. Her heart was racing, and she was very dizzy. Too late I discovered that the instructions on the prescription read three times per day rather than once per day. Fortunately, no harm came to her, and I corrected the error. But I was mortified. I had never—not one time—made an error of such magnitude in the days of handwritten prescriptions.

I soon came to view my role as protecting my patients from the EHR. I bet that that feature wasn't included in the sales pitch ("Ours is the least dangerous EHR."). But at least this gave doctors something else to complain about other than how hard it was to get paid! If anything, this was worse.

I was not alone. All around the nation, my experience was being replicated. Medical journals were filled with such stories.

A physician friend detailed his experiences using the popular EHR his health system purchased and distributed system-wide. In the days of paper charts, he used to finish most of his notes at the time of a visit. Now he can barely get them done the same day. This is such a problem in the health system that management had to initiate a policy requiring that all notes be completed within forty-eight hours of an appointment. His notes are transcribed using voice-recognition software, but he says that the system is so error prone that he has to spend a good deal of time reviewing the notes afterwards. He related a recent dictation where he stated that "the patient does *not* have a seizure disorder" but the software had missed the word "not"!

At least once per week, he gets an error message that closes the system and deletes a note or prescriptions that he had been entering. This has been happening more frequently of late. He, too, has cried when he lost a particularly long list of refills he had been working on!

A few years back, one of our local hospitals switched to a new and very well-known EHR. I only became aware of the change one day when I could no longer access my patients' records on their once-somewhat-functional web portal. No one had alerted me of the change. I contacted the hospital's well-staffed IT department to ask why I could no longer access the system. They could not figure it out. After a few days of calls to inquire about the issue, I spoke to one of my contacts in the hospital's public relations department. She told me that they were using a whole new system. The old system was gone. Shockingly, the IT department couldn't figure out this most basic issue.

Shortly thereafter, I was seeing a new patient who had an important respiratory problem. He just couldn't give me enough details about the issue for my satisfaction, so I called his pulmonologist to get more information. The pulmonologist's practice had recently switched, along with this hospital, to this new EHR.

The pulmonologist came to the phone and was very collegial. But the conversation we had was an odd one. I told him the patient's name and my clinical questions. He said, "Oh yes, I remember him. He's a really tall guy, right?" That was an odd question. The patient was of average height. The pulmonologist then asked, "He's an older guy, right?" This was another odd question.

Then the pulmonologist explained what was going on. He was using the new EHR, which, unfortunately, was not allowing him to view any of his patients' charts. So he was guessing! I did not need the information immediately, so we agreed we would speak in a few weeks, which we assumed would be enough time for the EHR to begin allowing him to actually see patient records again. Unfortunately, when I called back a few weeks later, he still could not access any of his patients' charts! Can you imagine how dangerous this was? I don't know how or why they continued to see patients under such circumstances.

I called the pulmonologist recently to get an update on his EHR experiences in the ensuing years. His practice had switched to a different product because of dissatisfaction with the original one. However, they still must use the original EHR in addition to the new one because their hospital still uses it. So, in essence, they are forced to maintain two sets of charts. However, their new system does not include their labs, so they also maintain paper charts for every patient. So, they actually have three parallel record systems! But they are not happy with their current system, either. At least once per day, the system locks up, and it takes considerable time to restart, forcing them, once again, to see patients without the benefit of their medical records! Just that day, he had seen a very ill patient and knew that the patient had just undergone testing that likely held crucial clues to what was wrong with them, but he could not get the results of the test because the system had shut down. He was forced to send the patient to the hospital. The practice is about to switch to another new system.

Release the Bureaucrats

Owing to such issues, by 2010 only a small percentage of physicians were using a full-fledged EHR. Many were just using components of an electronic system, such as an e-prescribing module. Into the fray jumped the federal government, whose role until that time had been essentially nonexistent. This had become a very big problem.

The bureaucrats of the Bush Administration era largely stayed out of medical computerization. Their belief was that the way forward should be determined by "the market." They believed in capitalism in an almost religious way—that financial and product markets moved like the unseen hand of God in determining the best way to develop health information technology. Unfortunately, what that meant was that a multitude of EHR systems now existed, each with its own data format, none of which could communicate with one another. Because there had been no real guidance regarding formatting or "interoperability," the capacity for these computer systems to communicate and share information with one another, each had gone in its own direction. We were stuck with a computerized Tower of Babel.

Further, the market for EHRs was the opposite of free. Systems tended to be so expensive that physician practices and health systems avoided them altogether, or if they did purchase a system, the investment of time and money was so great that purchasing a different system would be out of the question for years to come, no matter how they felt about their first EHR.

While the federal government understood there was a problem, their response ultimately made things much worse—our theme repeating itself once again. Enter the "Meaningful Use" program. Let me make myself clear. I cannot say enough bad things about this program, and I am not alone. Of the top ten challenges facing physicians identified in an annual survey by *Medical Economics*, Meaningful Use has been in the top four each of the last three years. Meaningful Use was poorly conceived and horribly executed. What has happened in the ensuing years leads me to question everything about the government bureaucracy that wields total power over our health-care system. If the federal government weren't so busy dirtying its diapers in so many other ways, the Meaningful Use program would be a huge scandal.

The idea underlying the Meaningful Use program was not a bad one. CMS wanted to increase EHR usage among US clinicians. They correctly surmised that excessive cost was one of the leading factors preventing doctors from adopting EHRs. They decided to subsidize the purchase. Understandably, they did not want to provide monetary incentives so that physicians could purchase just any system that could be used in just any way. So, in order to qualify for incentive payments, physicians were required to use EHR systems that had been certified according to Meaningful Use standards, and they had to show that they were using the systems "meaningfully," according to a list of specified criteria. All of this is okay as a general idea.

But the devil, as I have said before, is in the details. And the details of the Meaningful Use program make it a trap for unsuspecting doctors. EHRs are like running shoes. You don't know what they're like until you've gone running in them a few times. By then, they are yours. Most doctors, as it turned out, and most health systems and IT professionals, probably couldn't tell the difference between a good EHR and a bad one just from looking at it. Nor did they have much of a clue about implementing systems, the need for training, and a whole host of other issues that are essential to successful EHR use, even with a good system. Nor were they aware of the hidden costs most EHR purchases entailed. Despite that, the Meaningful Use program got them to take the leap, luring them into the trap with monetary incentives and then kicking them in from behind with financial penalties. They ended up purchasing systems that didn't work and then were required to jump through a multitude of silly government hoops and collect reams of inane government data with systems that, unfortunately, were not really designed for those purposes. Most doctors will tell you that the money wasn't worth the heartache. But by the time they figured that out, it was too late. And then the government changed its mind, sort of. Thanks, government.

The program debuted in 2011, offering a total of $44,000 per physician, spread over five years. I have to say, $44,000 excited me at first, as it was supposed to. It excited a lot of physicians. Health-system executives were more than excited by this money. If they multiplied $44,000 by the hundreds of physicians who worked for them, the dollar signs dancing in their heads made EHRs seem like crack cocaine. And this amount of money had its intended effect on many who, despite what they had heard about the downsides of

EHRs, finally took the plunge and purchased a system so that they could get their hands on the loot, too. As with crack, though, soon the regret sinks in.

Initially, the program was voluntary. Beginning in 2013, failure to participate began to carry penalties. That was an important aspect of the program, because once physicians began to understand the horrors of EHR systems, and then on top of that, the soul- and practice-crushing effects of the Meaningful Use program, if there hadn't been pretty significant carrots and sticks involved, nobody in their right mind would have participated.

Stage 1 of the Meaningful Use program was only terrible. I don't have words adequate to describe Stage 2 and the still-threatened Stage 3, but I will do my best.

So, to receive the monetary incentive that came with Meaningful Use Stage 1, there were fifteen required core measures. One of those required core measures was to report on at least six clinical quality measures, so the fifteen core measures were really twenty in total. Then there were ten additional "menu set" measures, from which you had to choose five. So, in total there were twenty-five requirements. To begin with, that's a lot of requirements. As usual, the bureaucrats who designed the program were unable to control themselves—and they went way too far.

Before you could attempt compliance with Meaningful Use, though, you had to learn about the program—but CMS made this almost impossible. The CMS website that I initially encountered for the Meaningful Use program was the worst website I have ever used. Finding the page that listed all the requirements, with each measure's details, was an exercise in mind-numbing futility. I found myself clicking promising links that only took me back to where I had been earlier, or took me to other pages that also had promising links that never seemed to give me the information I needed. It took me days to figure the program out.

If you could get past this Sisyphean website, you learned that some of the measures were not overly challenging, but, unfortunately, others were. The most basic measures tended to involve things that most physicians would consider fairly integral to good care. For instance, there were measures that specified that a patient record should include a "Problem list of current and active diagnoses," an "Active medication list," and a "Medical allergy list."

On the other hand, there were measures of dubious value that did nothing but create extra work and more clicks of the mouse. For instance, you were required to "Provide clinical summaries for patients for each office visit." So, at the end of each appointment, we had to prepare a summary that included, at a minimum, a problem list, results of any recent diagnostic tests, and a current medication and medication allergy list, in addition to advice specific to what had been discussed during that appointment.

I already provided my patients with similar "summaries," but I was doing it at my discretion when I thought it served a specific purpose and could be useful. But this measure required that it be done for 50 percent of all office appointments. It is debatable whether such summaries provide enough benefits to warrant requiring them 50 percent of the time (and to ensure meeting this threshold, many physicians gave them out 100 percent of the time). I can assure you that not every patient needs one or benefits from it. It was an unnecessary distraction and a significant waste of time. It also generated a good deal of paper. Ironically, one of the goals of computerization was to reduce the use of paper. Up to this point, my office had gone relatively paper free. Because of this Meaningful Use measure, there was more paper than ever!

Another measure requires that more than 10 percent "of all unique patients seen are provided patient-specific education resources." Many doctors like to give their patients information, such as educational handouts, when they think it might be helpful.

But to create a threshold requiring that we do this for 10 percent of office visits means that we just start giving patients handouts to satisfy the measure. There is very little data to show that providing this type of material improves clinical outcomes. And again, there was more paper being printed.

However, it was one matter to satisfy such silly measures, but a whole other issue to compile and report the data that demonstrated compliance. Not only did you have to provide patients with visit summaries and educational handouts, but in some EHRs, you also needed to remember to click a button to indicate that you had done so, enabling the EHR to register your work. That data then needed to be reported to CMS. These extra processes generated a substantial amount of work at the end of every appointment and quickly became another significant distraction.

One doctor told me, "I type things to satisfy the rules, and to get the money, but I'm losing time to talk to my patients and do things that really promote their well-being."

No measure is more maddening than one that requires us to "protect electronic health information through the implementation of appropriate technical capabilities." To comply, we must "conduct or review a security risk analysis in accordance with the requirements under 45 CFR 164.308(a)(1), including addressing the encryption/security of data stored in CEHRT in accordance with requirements under 45 CFR 164.312 (a)(2)(iv) and 45 CFR 164.306(d)(3), and implement security updates as necessary and correct identified security deficiencies as part of the provider's risk management process for EPs." Well that sounds simple enough, doesn't it? I'm kidding.

Fortunately, for those of us that don't know what rule 45 CFR 164.308(a)(1) is, the Meaningful Use website includes a link that takes you to an incomprehensible fifty-page excerpt from the Federal Register that describes the ruling. I can summarize this document for you in two words—don't bother. At one point, realizing that maybe they had made this measure just a tad cumbersome, CMS provided a tool to help doctors perform the required security review. I downloaded the tool only to find that it was composed of over six hundred questions, many of which I couldn't understand! Thanks, CMS.

Attestation, the official term for reporting Meaningful Use data, which is required each year in order to qualify for an incentive payment, is also far more difficult than you would expect. Attestation is accomplished through a maddering web portal. It only really involves answering a series of yes/no questions and entering numerical data. I don't even get how they make this difficult, but I can guarantee you, they have figured it out.

In one area of the attestation web portal, after having to enter both a numerical numerator and a denominator, they make *you* calculate the value of said numerator divided by the denominator and enter that value. Isn't that something that could be done by the computer? Isn't that just creating an opportunity to enter incorrect data where the computer could easily ensure that the data is correct by performing the calculation automatically?

In another area, after numerous screens that display the numerator on the left and the denominator on the right of a data entry line, they then switch, with the denominator on the left, and the numerator on the right. You begin to wonder if they are actually trying to make you mess this up!

Don't Worry, It Gets Worse

Suffice to say that this didn't go over real well in the medical community. But hey, there was money to be made and, of course, money to be lost, so who cares what the damn doctors thought?

And none of this changed the fact that EHRs were essentially unusable and still too expensive. It turned out that the combination of having to use horrible EHR technology and then additionally having to comply with this nutty Meaningful Use first stage was so confounding that doctors did not initially flock to do either. CMS's response to this situation was incredibly telling. In the good old-fashioned government way, rather than improving the Meaningful Use program (or even EHRs themselves), they created an entirely new industry to help administer this unholy hell. Enter the Regional Extension Centers (RECs), government-funded organizations intended to help doctors select and implement EHRs and comply with Meaningful Use.

Again, we see this horrible pattern. Rather than fix a bad situation (EHRs that are unusable) or improve burdensome and confusing regulations (insane Meaningful Use program), CMS creates a new layer of bureaucracy and administration.

And here's how this type of thing works. By 2013, after attesting for Meaningful Use two years in a row, with all the distractions, and extra mouse clicking, and all the printing of summaries and educational handouts, my friend and fellow physician Dr. Moyer (who is also founder of our EHR company, so we were using the same system) and I were both feeling a little burned out by the whole thing. We both loved our practices, and we loved our own dear EHR, but Meaningful Use was killing us.

So, Dr. Moyer contacted his state REC representative and asked if we could skip a year. He was told we could. We could skip a year and just resume the next year without incurring any penalty. So that's what we did. Except that advice was wrong. In 2015, because we had skipped 2013, we both received a 1 percent cut in the amount Medicare would pay us for any service we provided that year! We contacted that same REC representative, who now denied ever having told us we could skip the year. She even had the gall to ask if we had gotten this advice in writing. Unfortunately, we had trusted her since it was her job to know about these things and had not gone so far as to document her advice just in case she didn't know what the hell she was talking about. Now, I know that 1 percent isn't a large cut, but when it happens the way it did, it makes you insanely angry, let me assure you.

You think that was bad? CMS was just getting started. Before most doctors had completed Stage 1 of the Meaningful Use program, CMS announced Stage 2, and even threatened Stage 3. Well, Stage 1 was just the set-up punch. Stage 2 was the knockout blow.

So, what would you do if you had unusable technology and an overly complicated program intended to encourage more physicians to use that unusable technology in a specified but too complicated way? Of course, you would try to improve the technology and you would simplify the program. But CMS, apparently masters of reverse psychology, did the opposite.

Meaningful Use Stage 2 debuted in 2015. While many of the program's requirements remained unchanged, Stage 2 contained a number of new measures that made compliance essentially impossible for most physicians (and payments went down each year of participation in Meaningful Use, despite the increasing demands of the program). First of all, many EHR vendors were unable to provide the functionality (or get certified) to support Stage 2. If perchance your EHR was in compliance with Stage 2 requirements, then you likely had to pay to upgrade—all for the privilege of then having to try to do the ludicrous and the undoable.

For instance, to satisfy one of the measures in Stage 2, you have to get 5 percent of your patients to sign up to your online patient portal and 5 percent of your patients to send you an email using that portal. I spoke to a physician who described the silliness that transpired as a result of this new requirement. He said that, in an effort to achieve those 5 percent thresholds, 100 percent of the patients who have had an appointment (and who have an email account) receive an email afterward asking if they have any questions. Many patients respond with things like, "No I don't have any questions, but thanks for asking." The physician who saw that patient then receives that message, to which they must respond! So, doctors, who are already overburdened with a combination of clinical responsibilities and burgeoning administrative demands, now also have to respond to inane emails every day on top of everything else! Do you see why I called this book *Distracted*?

Even better, now 10 percent of your referrals to outside providers had to be done via email through a special secure communications portal. We encountered a slight problem with this measure, though, as literally none of our referral colleagues had such a portal! My staff spent hours contacting other offices to get their new "secure" email addresses. Most of the offices had no idea what we were referring to. None of them had one of these special email addresses!

Meaningful Use Stage 2 was essentially dead on arrival. The negative response was so overwhelming that in March 2015, recognizing that only a tiny percentage of clinicians could or would participate, CMS announced it was putting the program on temporary hold while it reorganized. The message was, essentially, "We'll get back to you sometime." They hinted at a number of changes, including that data collection requirements would be reduced for 2015 from a whole year down to ninety days. Then things got really quiet—for a long time.

Here's where things really get good, though. CMS didn't get back to us until October 6, 2015. Now, I've made it clear that I'm just a simple country doctor, and certainly no math expert, but it seems to me that if you need to collect ninety days of data for the year, but they don't even tell you what that data is until there are roughly only eighty-four days left in the year, there is a problem. Not to mention the small fact that every existing EHR needed to retool their systems to reflect the new measures and reporting requirements of this new version of Stage 2 Meaningful Use, and then had to train physicians how to use these retooled systems, as well. I swear I am not making this up.

One other fun fact is that in addition to this nightmare of unbelievable incompetence, on October 1, CMS was also forcing the entire medical nation to switch to a brand-new set of diagnostic codes. This switch, from the ICD-9 diagnosis code set to ICD-10, had been canceled the prior year, so no way was CMS going to look more stupid than it already did and cancel it again. Just to put this into some perspective—medical practice management consultants were regularly advising that practices have six months of operating cash on hand because glitches in implementing this changeover could potentially hold up payments for that long! Certainly we could go six months without getting paid—who couldn't?

Of course, you would expect that they would coordinate things better than to schedule these two incredibly profound, essentially life-altering changes at the same time, because if you combine two impossible changes, the potential risks of calamity would be unacceptable—except that's exactly what they did.

Still, it gets better! You could probably count on two hands the number of physicians who were able to comply with this new unimproved Stage 2 Meaningful Use (I happened to be one of them, but I don't like to brag).

Things were so fouled up by this point that CMS granted a special hardship exemption for physicians who could not comply with Meaningful Use in 2015, so they could avoid what was now a 3 percent Medicare payment penalty. Recognizing that just about every breathing physician was going to apply for this hardship, CMS made the exemption easier to apply for and then even extended the deadline.

And then the nuclear bomb dropped. On January 11, 2016, one Andy Slavitt, who happens to be the CMS acting administrator, while at the J.P. Morgan Health Care Conference in Las Vegas, announced, "The Meaningful Use program, as it has existed, will now be effectively over and replaced with something better." A more cynical person than me might say, "Pretty much anything could be better," but I wouldn't do that.

This was, of course, pretty big news, but I wasn't sure whether to cheer or to cry. My first thought was actually to wonder why this announcement was made at the J.P. Morgan Health Care Conference, described as "the biggest health-care investing event of the year," and not made directly to physicians, who have been suffering at the hands of this stupid program? Again, if I were cynical about these things, I might surmise that Big Money had stopped getting big enough returns on Meaningful Use and therefore needed to be placated with something new.

If it were true that Meaningful Use was actually dead and gone, I would cheer. But with CMS's record, can we assume that it would be replaced by something better? I don't know why we would. On the other hand, my EHR company had just spent $26,000 becoming certified for Stage 2 Meaningful Use! If Meaningful Use was canceled, could we get our damn money back?

But let's not get ahead of ourselves. It appears that when a government official says that Meaningful Use "will now be effectively over," he means something other than "will now be effectively over." Eight days later, Mr. Slavitt "clarified" his original statement, saying that physicians will still be required to attest to the criteria of Meaningful Use using certified health-record technology. Don't worry, physicians learned to stop trusting CMS a long time ago.

Where We Are Today

The most basic problem is that most EHR technology is not yet ready for prime time. Most EHR systems are largely unusable, cost too much, and do little to improve the quality of medical care. As the information in this section has shown, in many ways their implementation has made medical care worse and less safe.

Lack of guidance from the federal government was an early problem. When they tried to right the ship, they made things much worse. They made far too many demands—demands that changed almost constantly—of technology that was not up to the task.

Their system of incentives and penalties essentially forced a generation of medical professionals to commit professional suicide by purchasing EHR technology whose expense and technical challenges prevent moving to something better, if and when that comes along.

A September 2016 article in *U.S. News and World Report* titled "Do Electronic Health Records Breed Burnout?" reported on a survey that sums up the current state of affairs. "'The clerical burden associated with electronic health records has been a major contributing factor to physician burnout,' says Dr. Tait Shanafelt, the lead author of a study on the issue and director of the Mayo Clinic Department of Medicine Program on Physician Well-Being." Their study found that "nearly half of US doctors are burned out, and many believe electronic health records, or EHRs, are partly to blame. . . . The tools now on the market have failed to live up to expectations. . . . They have generated widespread exasperation among physicians, with 44 percent of respondents who used electronic health records reporting that they were dissatisfied or very dissatisfied with them. Forty-one percent disagreed or strongly disagreed with the notion that the records have improved patient care."

When asked about this study's results, the new director of the Office of the National Coordinator for Health Information Technology (ONC), Virdell Washington, MD, could only say, "It's an area of change. Technology will evolve. . . . At the end of the day, keeping your eye on having improved patient outcomes and better patient care, the efficiencies, I believe, will follow." In other words, he doesn't get it, he doesn't much care, and things aren't going to be changed.

Physicians are stuck in the middle of a terrible predicament between a technology that they do not understand and can't control, and a bureaucratic machine that will not stop and that has no rudder. So, if at some point you are at the doctor's office and you are trying to get some important point through to your physician, who happens to be sitting in front of the computer, and she has an odd, or even horrified, look on her face and seems to be just a bit distracted, now you know why! That computer is the abyss, and she is staring into it!

In an op-ed published in the September 22, 2016, issue of the *Wall Street Journal*, two physicians, Caleb Gardner, MD, and John Levinson, MD, lamented, "Not long ago, doctors dreamed of a time when unwieldy paper charts would be replaced by streamlined computer systems, freeing them up for more direct patient care. But now these computer systems are distracting and burdensome. Senior physicians are retiring early because of the EHR, while young doctors feel the humanity draining from a profession to which many were drawn because of a desire to interact and connect with people."

All told, billions of dollars of both private and public money have been wasted on what has been an astounding debacle. More than $23.5 billion in Medicare EHR Incentive Program payments have been made between May 2011 and 2016. More than $10.9 billion in Medicaid EHR Incentive Program payments have been made between January 2011 (when the first set of states launched their programs) and June 2016. But most physicians will tell you that the money they received wasn't worth the trouble they have been through, and continue to go through, using systems that still cost too much, don't do what they need to be done, and keep them working into the night trying to catch up. The most promising change in the history of medicine has gone almost entirely unfulfilled, and administrative and bureaucratic mismanagement is almost entirely to blame. On top of that, physician stress and the distractions directly related to EHR use are immense. More than any single issue, this one must be fixed if we want real improvements in the American health-care system.

The Fix

Stop everything! Every current government project that involves computers and medicine should be suspended or stopped right now.

Stop it all so that doctors can recover and refocus their efforts and their energies back on patient care. Stop it all until there is an affordable system that can do what we ask of it. CMS should very publicly and very clearly announce a consistent ten-year plan for health-care computerization that includes standards for functionality, usability, and interoperability, and then hold a one- or two-year competition to create such a system.

When that system becomes available, and only then, CMS should use public funds to offer the software very affordably or even free to every physician practice and health system in the nation. It should be available both through the cloud and on local servers, so that practices in locations without dependable Internet service can use the system.

As a part of interoperability, data mining and aggregation should be completely automated so that any data from the system can be collected without any work for health-care providers, who should be able to refocus on patient care, aided by a functional computer system rather than tortured by it.

The system should be so robust that it can be implemented and maintained with a minimum of IT support and personnel.

Operation, support, and training should be thorough and comprehensive and should be available through a functional centralized website. That way, everyone can be knowledgeable about the system, and use of the system will be as consistent as possible.

I guarantee this can be done. It absolutely must be done.

CHAPTER 5

Your Health Insurance May Kill You

U p until now, I've primarily been going after government
bureaucrats. But in the introductory section, I said it was
government bureaucrats *and* health insurance executives
who were the problem. So, to be fair, I thought I would start in on
these executives now.

We can debate the reasons and the solutions, but the fact is
that having insurance as the financial hub of our health-care system is not working. Many millions of people don't have insurance,
and many who have insurance are decimated financially as a direct
result. But worse still, many people who have insurance still do not
receive the care they need or pay large amounts when they do. It is a
deep moral stain in a country where many of the citizens believe that
what goes on is supposed to reflect their Christian values. We argue
incessantly, and even kill one another, over the value of life, but the
reality is that when a patient's life is on the line because of illness,
health insurance often just doesn't give a damn. And we can also
argue about what is worst about American health care, but health

insurance is inarguably its cruelest aspect, because it denies care that would otherwise be readily available to those who need it.

Having health insurance was once the equivalent of having health care. But that is no longer the case. Having health insurance guarantees only one thing—having to pay the premiums. Aside from that, having health insurance no longer means you have access to health care—and that is a very big problem. This is an obvious problem for patients, but it affects health professionals as well, both in terms of their ability to care for patients and their approaches in delivering this care. And it is one more distraction in a rising sea of them.

Our Love Affair with Health Insurance

Most of us became aware of health care as an important political issue in the 1990s, when the Clintons, two people from Arkansas, made fixing the health-care industry their top priority. Bill Clinton staked the early part of his presidency on the issue and came away with nothing. Fortunately, other scandals distracted us from that fact, and, in this respect, his reputation remained intact.

At that time, the issue of greatest concern was the rising cost of health care. It seems almost comical now, but health care accounted for about 8 percent of the gross domestic product then, a figure that elicited dread the way that ISIS does today. It was feared that if health expenditures continued to grow unabated, they would begin to affect our ability to pay for anything else. Health-care spending stands at close to 18 percent of GDP today.

Doctors are not immune to the ravages of the health insurance system when they become patients. I thought that when I became a doctor, maybe I got a membership to a secret club that included free health care as one of its perks. It is symbolic, then, that I actually needed the health-care system for the first time as an adult during my first year of medical school, when I broke my wrist quite badly. Not to worry, my wife and I thought, we have health insurance, and this is the greatest health-care system in the world.

We went to the ER, where the break was diagnosed and a splint applied. I was given an appointment to see an orthopedic surgeon. The next day, that orthopedic surgeon told us that I had to leave and go to my primary care doctor first. I had never seen my "primary care doctor" before, but nonetheless, we went to the office listed on my insurance card. But they informed me that the orthopedist I had seen was not in-network, so they directed us to a different orthopedist. I saw him the next day, and he was very nice, but he informed me that he didn't work on wrists. So, it was back to the primary care office, where they gave us an appointment with orthopedist number three, who, fortunately, did work on wrists. After five days and visits to four different medical offices thanks to our confusing insurance, I finally got the surgery to repair the break. But despite our fine health insurance, a few months later I had the pleasure of receiving a $400 bill. It turned out that one of the doctors that had taken care of me in the hospital wasn't in-network. So, why did he see me, we wondered?

It was an eye-opening experience. This was the greatest health care in the world? At least back then, even though we were getting screwed, we weren't paying much for the insurance that was doing it. Today, you get screwed *and* you pay Eliot Spitzer prices.

In 2000, when I began my first job as a physician at a public health clinic, one of the impressive selling points of the job was that the health insurance there was free to the employees—that's right, free! It makes my head swim just thinking about it. It almost seems comical how shocked we felt a couple of years later when management announced that, for the first time, we would have to pay a portion of our insurance costs. Like everyone else, we soon became used to annual increases, sometimes huge increases, in our premiums.

This was a walk in the park, though, compared to what we experienced in 2009, when I opened my own medical practice, and for the first time, my family was shopping for health insurance on the open market. Apparently, I had been rather spoiled up until that point. We knew that doctors could purchase health insurance through the Maryland State medical association. They happily referred me to their insurance representative, who informed me that we could get insurance for the small fee of $2,500. I actually had to ask, "Per month?" Yes, per month. Thanks, but no thanks. We went elsewhere. Despite our best efforts, by the end of the decade, my healthy family of three was paying $800 per month for our health insurance, and our policy carried a $10,000 deductible. In other words, even with insurance, the first $20,000 of any health-related catastrophe was ours to pay!

At least we could take comfort in the fact that we were in good company. Horror stories about the costs of health care in America had become the norm. By 2010, medical costs were the number one cause of personal bankruptcy in the United States. Many of those who had insurance were paying exorbitant prices. Worse still, close to 50 million people were without any health insurance at all.

More and more, we were seeing the heartbreaking effects of our fraying medical system in practice. Federally Qualified Health Centers (FQHCs), government-supported primary care clinics, where I spent the early part of my career, received an explosion in funding in the early 2000s in response to the rising number of uninsured Americans. Rather than fixing the system, they were just one more Band-Aid on the gaping wound. Even with billions of dollars in new funding and new FQHCs springing up all over the country, this could not meet the need.

It was hard to believe, but I had more than one tough uninsured patient perform their own skin surgeries rather than face the cost of seeing a surgeon. And I vividly remember talking to one woman who needed a gynecologic surgery. My office was just a few blocks from a shiny new hospital where the surgery could be performed, but at a cost to her of $10,000 that she did not have. She ended up traveling to the Dominican Republic, where for $2,000 she received the surgery, had a prolonged hospital stay, and then spent another month visiting family in the country. She was one of the lucky ones. Around the same time, I saw a woman who had been complaining of abdominal pain for much of the past year but had not been able to afford the costs of testing to evaluate her problem. When finally her family had scraped together enough money for her abdominal CT scan, the cancer we found was advanced and it was too late.

This was the disturbing health-care experience in the wealthiest nation the world had ever known. In 2009, it was estimated that there were forty-five thousand deaths in the United States related to lack of health insurance. And this was the best health care in the world? It was more than obvious that things were not working. Enter Obamacare.

Obama to the Rescue

Let's give credit to everyone who deserves it—President Obama for having the balls and the naïve enthusiasm to try and fix health care against all odds, and the insurance and pharmaceutical companies for being so damned crafty as to fool everybody into thinking that they might actually go along with it!

No one in their right mind at the time was hopeful about the chances of health-care reform. Coming off the financial disaster of 2008, it seemed like a pretty steep mountain the president was trying to climb, and I don't remember anyone else in the Democratic leadership acting very excited about helping him. And, of course, every congressional Republican was busy doing everything he or she could think of to undermine the effort (except propose anything better).

Senator Max Baucus, the Montana Democrat who was chairman of the Senate Finance Committee responsible for writing the Affordable Care Act, looked absolutely ashen throughout the process. He had taken literally millions of dollars in campaign contributions from the insurance industry in the years running up to his work on Obamacare, so I guess he was in a difficult position. I often wondered what Obama had on him to get him to push for the few changes that he did eventually advocate. On the other hand, he forbade discussion of a single-payer option or the health insurance public option, and allowed insurance company lobbyists to write entire sections of the Obamacare law, so I think he satisfied his funders. But he was so traumatized by his experience that he retired from the Senate in 2014. He was then given the ambassadorship to China, a country which does, ironically, have universal health care. But they also force everyone to have their colonoscopies.

The initial rollout of Obamacare was a nightmare of historic proportions. Initially, the federal government and many state governments were unable to successfully construct the websites that were to be the online marketplaces where people would purchase their new health insurance policies. So, for months, few people could actually sign up for Obamacare. This astonishing show of incompetence was one of the most embarrassing moments in the history of American government. Throw in a couple of government shutdowns and a historic level of partisanship and gridlock to boot, and many Americans have completely lost faith in the United States' ability to govern. The online insurance exchanges were slowly repaired, but the debacle pushed Obamacare to the brink of collapse.

Hyperpolarization was nowhere more apparent than in the congressional reaction to Obamacare. The Republican leadership and pundits hate Obamacare because of Obama. The Republicans almost unanimously call for Obamacare's repeal. They would replace it with—really nothing. Most Democrats not named Obama initially went into hiding over Obamacare, but now sort of point to its success. They say things like "Obamacare is not perfect, but we must build on its successes " This is in contrast to famed liberal economist and *New York Times* columnist Paul Krugman, who gushes uncontrollably about Obamacare no matter what.

But let's cut to the chase. Is Obamacare a success? The answer is a little complicated, but it's no. Here is my brief analysis.

First and foremost, when President Obama caved on the inclusion of a public option, a basic health insurance policy provided by the government that would have, ostensibly, been priced affordably and would have offered a package of reasonable care, Obamacare was doomed. Presumably, the public option would have established the baseline with which the insurance industry would have had to compete. The insurance industry argued that it could not compete, and it won. This gave them carte blanche to uphold the status quo. Obamacare was crippled as a result.

Second, the legislation was just too voluminous. The bill came in at around 2,700 pages, and there are now 20,000 pages of regulations associated with it. I haven't read the bill, our legislators haven't read it, and you haven't read it. Its excessive size and complexity doom it to the confusion and misinterpretation that is the hallmark of bad bureaucracy.

Access to Medical Care: More May Be Less

President Obama is most proud of the ACA's effects on expanding and improving health insurance coverage. The number of uninsured individuals in the United States has declined from 49 million in 2010 to 29 million in 2015. Obamacare has clearly provided health insurance to many people who could not get insurance previously.

So, Obamacare is approaching 50 percent success in providing health insurance to people who did not have it before. When

President Obama and pundits like Krugman call Obamacare a success, they are usually referring to this fact, as well as a purported slowdown in health-care spending increases. As I previously stated, though, having health insurance is no longer equivalent to having medical care. As with everything else we have discussed in this book, the devil is in the details.

Once people were actually able to access the exchanges and purchase insurance, things improved for some people, at least temporarily. There were four clear benefits from Obamacare. First and foremost, some people who could not get health insurance, and therefore care, got both. Second was the fact that children of insured parents could remain on their parents' policies until the age of twenty-six. Third was the elimination of previously existing conditions as a means for disqualifying people from receiving insurance. And finally, certain preventive services had to be offered to patients at no cost.

After that, the effects become murky. First of all, many people still do not have health insurance. Twenty-nine million uninsured is still a very large number. Second, many people still have health insurance policies that are exceedingly expensive. And third, many Obamacare-era health insurance policies contain provisions that effectively prevent them from receiving health care. So, *we traded millions of uninsured people for millions who are insured but can't get care.* Despite President Obama's rationalizations, this most important aspect of Obamacare represents continued failure to a significant extent.

A case in point is the many people who obtained their new policies through state Medicaid programs, which lowered their income eligibility criteria markedly. On the plus side, these new policies are heavily subsidized and therefore are usually affordable for those who qualify. On the negative side, though, Medicaid policies often pay so little to physicians that many will not accept them. So, despite now being insured, many people still find it difficult to find physicians who will care for them.

But when Obamacare debuted in 2014, the new Medicaid insurance policies were accompanied by a helpful wrinkle that obscured this problem temporarily. With the help of federal subsidies that were provided in 2014 and 2015, state Medicaid insurance programs were able to pay physicians Medicare rates, which are typically much higher. For a practice like mine, which had always accepted Medicaid patients out of moral obligation, finally getting paid decently for our efforts seemed like an incredible boon.

Unfortunately, after two years, those subsidies went away, and many states were then forced to dramatically lower what they paid. West Virginia, which accounted for many of my practice's new Medicaid patients, announced that it would be cutting payments by 50 percent. Because of this, and a number of other factors which will be detailed momentarily, we stopped accepting new West Virginia Medicaid patients. We continued to see previously established West Virginia Medicaid patients despite the losses. For our efforts, we were rewarded in the spring of 2016 with a letter that read, "As you are aware, the state faces a significant deficit for fiscal year 2016 which is also projected to continue into fiscal year 2017. Absent an upward trend in revenues or a funding solution identified, the Bureau for Medical Services will be unable to process claims at the same consistent level that has been maintained." In other words, we were now being informed that if we continued to see West Virginia Medicaid patients, it might have to be for free!

Under such circumstances, it is hard to imagine that many of the people who have obtained these new health insurance policies in the Obamacare era will find that medical care is any more accessible than it was when they had no insurance in the previous era.

For those who did not qualify for Medicaid under Obamacare, it has also been a mixed bag. Many people, my family included, were initially able to purchase health insurance for less than they had been paying previously. But this was also a temporary situation for many (again, my family included).

The health insurance industry has proven over the years that, if nothing else, it is a survivor. And to survive, it will do whatever it takes. During the initial debates over Obamacare's enactment, the PR against health insurers, whom most people view as being somewhere between dirty toilets and pepper spray to the eyes, was horrible. The Affordable Care Act was gaining critical mass, and in order to survive, industry executives gave in on a number of fronts, enabling Obamacare to move forward. They understood that failure to play ball at all would have brought about consideration of a single-payer option, which could have eliminated commercial health insurance altogether.

Then, when it was initially reported that health insurance premiums for Obamacare policies on the whole had not skyrocketed as feared, many pointed to this as a sign of Obamacare's impending success. When, in year two, most health insurance premiums remained steady, it began to appear that President Obama might be on to something.

But I believe that this was all part of a very carefully orchestrated insurance industry plan—play nice for a few years and then begin to turn the screws again. As President Obama very blandly states in a 2016 *JAMA* article, "both insurers and policy-makers are still learning about the dynamics of an insurance market that includes all people regardless of any preexisting conditions, and further adjustments and recalibrations will likely be needed, as can be seen in some insurers' proposed Marketplace premiums for 2017."

In other words, premiums are back on their way up. "For states that have made their 2017 requests public, insurers are making hefty premium requests. In North Carolina, the largest insurer, Blue Cross, is seeking an 18.8 percent increase for 2017, while Aetna is seeking 24.5 percent, and United Healthcare is withdrawing entirely. Insurers in other states, such as New York and Georgia, are attempting to raise rates by 20 percent or more," reports a June 2016 blog post for Zane Benefits, which specializes in individual health insurance reimbursement for small businesses. Obamacare defenders say that premiums would have gone up even more had it not been the law of the land. But it is little solace to the millions of Americans who struggle to afford health care to say, "Hey, it could have been worse."

Insurance for Insurers' Profits

But that's just the beginning. Health insurance companies have begun to use four other profit-ensuring tools with far more abandon: deductibles, prior authorization requirements, restrictive prescription formularies, and incomplete coverage. You have to hand it to these insurance companies, they're good at what they do, by which I mean making money at our expense.

Significant deductibles, which were not something we heard much about a decade ago, are becoming increasingly common. The percentage of workers with a general annual deductible has increased from 55 percent in 2006 to 81 percent in 2015. And the average deductible amount has risen 255 percent over that same time. So, in addition to having to deal with rising premiums, if you actually need health care, your out-of-pocket expenses are rising as well. This has two obvious effects. It protects and increases insurance company profits, and it limits patients' ability to get medical care. As a result, I now regularly have patients who have health insurance but are unable to afford tests or treatments.

Nationwide, nearly 30 percent of people insured through the federal marketplace who had deductibles higher than $1,500 went without needed medical care in 2014 because they could not afford it, according to Families USA, a health-care consumer group based in Washington, DC. A September 2016 article in the *Washington Post*, titled "How companies are quietly changing your health plan to make you pay more," reported on a study by the Health Care Cost Institute analyzing insurance claims data between 2010 and 2014. They found that people with high-deductible plans used 10 percent fewer health-care services. The study also showed that despite that, these people paid significantly more on out-of-pocket expenses ($1,030) than people in more traditional plans ($687). So, people with high-deductible insurance pay more to get less. Many economists consider this a good thing—people with "skin in the game" will "cut back on unnecessary care if they are on the hook for more of the costs." But I can assure you, they avoid necessary care as well, and they suffer as a result.

In addition, insurers have begun to institute more and more onerous prior authorization requirements. Prior authorization means that when a doctor orders a test or a drug, it first has to be approved by the insurance company through processes that can take just minutes in some instances, but might also take hours or even days.

I recently saw a patient who complained of a pulsing sound in the right ear and of losing balance and falling to that same side. These are symptoms that could be the harbinger of a life-threatening brain aneurysm. I appropriately ordered a magnetic resonance angiogram of the head. It took my nurse an hour on the phone with the insurance company, first on one call to get an accession number (an official number for the request), and once she had obtained that, on a second call to present the "clinicals" (the facts of the case that justify the request). Then a physician came on the line for a "peer-to-peer" review of the same information with me. The test was approved, but only after this time-consuming process.

The problem is that we are already overburdened by stupid administrative tasks that detract from our ability to complete our clinical work. But also, we shy away from ordering necessary tests or treatments because we know that either they won't get approved or the work to get them approved will be too onerous. Even worse, we have stopped accepting patients with certain insurances that we know have the worst prior authorization requirements.

In the earliest days of Obamacare, I had a patient with a newly minted Obamacare policy who came in with symptoms of a possible stroke. It was not an immediate emergency because the symptoms had begun days before. Still, I thought a CT scan or an MRI of his head was necessary under the circumstances, and I thought it should be done quickly. Other possible diagnoses included things like a bleed in the brain or a brain tumor, so it was reasonable to want the testing and for the testing to be done quickly. It was a no brainer! Get it?

As I remember, we saw the patient about mid-morning on a Friday, and I asked my staff to have the test done that day, which had normally been possible in the past. We contacted one of the local radiology services, and they confirmed that they could indeed perform the test that day. Unfortunately, the patient's new policy required prior authorization for such things. My staff tried for hours to get the okay, but to no avail. They called the approval line but had to wait on call for a prolonged period of time. Then they presented the patient's demographic information to one person, and the clinical facts of the case to another. They answered a clinical questionnaire. They were placed on hold for long periods of time, multiple times. The case then went for clinical review. I spoke to someone about mid-afternoon, and as my nurses had already done, explained the rationale and need for the testing. At 5:10 that evening, hearing my nurses still on the phone trying to get the test approved, I got on the phone and loudly registered my irritation at the delay, foul language included. I never would have done such a thing in the past (and I had never had to), but I have developed the skill out of necessity. Finally, someone came on the line who said that the test seemed reasonable. Which is why I had ordered it. The MRI did, in fact, reveal that our patient had experienced a small stroke.

After a number of similar experiences with this company, and then also finding that the same barriers made it difficult to refer our patients to specialists and that many specialists didn't accept this insurance anyway, we dropped this insurer.

Another fun trick the insurance companies use is incomplete coverage. Many people are still unfamiliar with this tactic. What I mean by incomplete coverage is that, even after you take out a second mortgage to pay your premiums and deductible, health insurance still doesn't always cover the care you receive or require. The problem is that you may not actually discover it until you get the bill months after you've left the hospital.

So, for instance, we had a very nice family—the whole family was insured—who had the great misfortune of having one of their children become quite ill with an E. coli infection that nearly caused kidney failure, which can happen in rare circumstances. They were thankful, and so were we, that they had good insurance, because we ended up sending the child to Children's Hospital in Washington, DC. Fortunately, our young patient recovered fully. The only problem was that sometime later the family received a bill for $30,000! It turned out that some of the treating physicians at the hospital were not covered by their insurance. But hey, who doesn't have a spare $30,000 lying around? The patient's mother recently told me that they are still making payments on this bill. More and more, my patients report similar stories. Some of them have waged small administrative wars to fight (and sometimes reduce or eliminate) similar charges that they felt were in error. But who wants (or has the will to fight) such hassles when they are ill?

I don't want to sound negative when it comes to Obamacare, so I will only discuss one more of its shortfalls. When they first announced the health insurance exchanges, they made it sound like these would be online marketplaces where we could pick and choose among various insurance options based on relative costs and benefits, and other such things—although you really just choose the cheapest one because even that you can't really afford. Well, guess what? In our region of the fine state of West Virginia, the only choice we get is Highmark Blue Cross Blue Shield. That's it. That is not a robust list of choices. This is becoming much more common. In August 2016, there were seven states that have only one issuer: Alabama, Alaska, Oklahoma, South Carolina, Wyoming, Kansas, and North Carolina. Large sections of other states, including Florida, Utah, and Missouri, may also be down to one carrier. There is even a county in Arizona where there may be no carriers in the marketplace.

One Patient's Experience in the Era of Obamacare

Frank, a longtime patient who has diabetes, described his harrowing experience with health care in the era of Obamacare. Frank took early retirement in March 2014 and began drawing social security benefits. He lost his health insurance when he retired. He took a part-time job in April 2014 for added income and then went to full-time hours in July 2014. His new employer offered health insurance that ran over $700 per month, but he was unable to afford that amount. Unfortunately, in January 2015, Frank was hospitalized. This cost him $15,000, which he paid. Then, between January and March 2015, Frank was fined by the government for not having health insurance.

In April 2015, Frank obtained insurance through the ACA marketplace. He currently has a policy that costs about $500 per month. After filing his federal taxes in 2015, he was notified by the IRS that the subsidy he had received to help pay for his insurance had been too high, and he was forced to give back $1,267. Also, because Frank earned more than $15,800 in 2015, he had to return approximately $4,500 of his social security benefits. Consequently, he cut back to part-time hours again, but is earning $10,000 less per year, which makes it a struggle to pay the premium for his new health insurance.

But at least he has insurance, right? Wrong. As a result of his diabetes, Frank has neuropathy, a painful condition affecting his feet. He saw a podiatrist regularly, as do many patients with this condition. With his new insurance, his portion of any specialist visit is a $30 co-pay. However, after each visit to the podiatrist, Frank received a bill between $50 and $80. His insurance refused to cover this, and he had to pay.

The podiatrist recommended that Frank purchase a special pair of shoes to protect his feet. He was told that his insurance covered the shoes, which would cost $150. Frank was wary, so he asked them to verify that the shoes were covered, which they did, multiple times. After receiving the shoes, Frank received a bill from the podiatrist. The shoes had not been covered. The bill Frank received was for $400, the actual amount the podiatrist was billing the insurance company! Frank has appealed the claim, but to no avail. When he refused to pay the bill, he was told to return the shoes, after he had worn them for six months!

Frank's new health insurance does include coverage for most prescriptions. However, he is no longer able to get his medications through our local pharmacy, where he has gone for many years. He is instead required to get them through a Walgreens thirty-five miles away. But not all of his prescriptions are covered. Frank has a nut allergy and was even hospitalized after a bad reaction in 2004. He has since carried an EpiPen—but no longer. When Mylan Pharmaceuticals raised the price of the EpiPen to an outlandish $600, he could no longer afford this lifesaving medication.

As a final affront, Frank's new employer is facing a fine because, purportedly, the policy they offered Frank (that he was unable to afford) did not meet ACA standards, forcing Frank to purchase his policy through the marketplace. His employer claims the policy met the standard and is appealing the fine, as well as Frank's decision not to purchase what he felt he could not afford.

Frank told me, "I am being forced to overpay for insurance that doesn't work, in a system that pits me against my employer, and I am fined if I make enough to afford the insurance." He says that his number one worry is the cost of his health insurance. He is worried that he will lose his job over these issues.

Of course, we know that Frank is not alone. As a result of Obamacare, a significant number of Americans are now required to purchase a product many of them can't afford, and for which they may receive little if any benefit—especially not peace of mind. We used to think of health insurance as something that protected us from financial disaster. Now it does more to protect health insurance company profits than anything else. The only reasonable conclusion we can draw is that the current system is just not working.

Practicing Medicine in the Era of Obamacare

Until now, we have been discussing Obamacare primarily as it affects patients. Patients are important, and some say, should even be the focus of our health-care system, so this discussion has not been unimportant. But let's remember that this is a book about how regulation is destroying the practice of medicine. It turns out that high deductibles, the need for prior authorizations, tight prescription formularies, and incomplete coverage also affect a physician's ability to practice medicine. In fact, Obamacare-era health insurance policies often dictate an entirely new approach to medical care—an approach that is far more complicated, and even at times more expensive, than medical care of the previous era.

In many ways, trying to take care of patients with newer insurance policies is a lot like it was taking care of people who didn't have health insurance at all. There are just a lot more nuances, or shall we say, distractions. It is a particular challenge to evaluate and treat patients who often can't afford evaluation or treatment.

With uninsured patients, things are relatively simple. The question is merely what someone can or cannot afford. Of course, with 29 million people remaining uninsured, we are still dealing with this with annoying frequency.

With Obamacare-era health insurance, access to care depends on what patients are able to afford, various insurance idiosyncrasies, and knowledge of the necessary workarounds that medical professionals need in order to deal with both. This entails a whole new set of skills that, unfortunately, are not taught in medical schools. In fact, I have identified at least four new models of medical care that have come into existence in the Obamacare era: the Workaround; the Lie; the Bargain; and the You Better Find Something Wrong with Me.

The Workaround

A Workaround is a special process that someone in my office has to figure out in order to obtain a test or medication for a patient. My staff is particularly adept at Workarounds. In recent years, they have had to develop a whole new set of skills and an entirely new knowledge base in order to obtain care for our patients. Unfortunately, this can take a lot of extra work, as we have discussed. But it also means that some patients may not receive the care they need unless they have a physician whose staff is smart enough, cares enough, and just has the time to figure out and execute these Workarounds.

A recent case will help to illustrate one such Workaround. A patient who has recurrent lung cancer began to experience progressively worsening pain of the lower abdomen, which then spread to the chest, the upper shoulders, the middle of the back, and the right arm. It didn't take a genius to know that this pain could indicate that the cancer was spreading. But it might take a genius to obtain the testing that could prove or disprove this diagnosis in the era of Obamacare.

The patient reported this pain to his oncologist, who ordered an MRI of the spine to look for the cause of the pain. I was confused about this order, though, because this test would only partially visualize the painful areas. If we didn't look further, we might miss the source of the pain.

I also knew there was a much better test in such circumstances— a PET scan. A PET scan is used specifically to identify cancerous growth and would visualize the patient's entire body. It was clearly the best test under the circumstances. Unfortunately, PET scans are also tough to obtain because insurance companies have arduous prior authorization processes that often block, or at least significantly delay, the test. But I guessed that an oncologist would have a much easier time of getting this test approved since he is a specialist.

With all this in mind, I picked up the phone and called the oncologist to see if I could talk him into ordering the PET scan. He was happy that I had called because the case was becoming increasingly complicated, and this would be a chance for us to better coordinate our care. He thought he needed to get an MRI first in order to justify the PET scan to the insurance company. This is a typical Workaround. He agreed that the PET scan was the most appropriate test but didn't think it would get approved without first getting the MRI. But I have a lot of faith in my staff, so we decided to let my staff try to get the PET scan approved. Shockingly, it was. I called the oncologist, who was surprised by the news. He canceled the MRI.

See how damn complicated it gets just to obtain necessary testing? It takes extra phone calls and hours of extra work to take care of the patient. Had we ended up getting the MRI, it would have added a substantial cost, as well (an MRI of the low back in our area costs approximately $1,200).

But that was nothing compared to this next Workaround. Not long ago we received the heartbreaking news that a patient whom we had known and taken care of for many years (and maybe it doesn't need to be said, but about whom we cared a great deal) had developed a heroin addiction and overdosed and very nearly died the day before. It was essential that we get the patient into detox and rehab immediately to prevent the possible tragedy that might occur when they used again. Fortunately, the patient had insurance, and the family was committed to scraping together as much money as they could to help with any uncovered expenses.

My nurse, Lindy, contacted the insurer's mental-health prior-authorization department. She presented the details of the case. The insurance approved a brief stay for detox at a local hospital. But we knew that this hospital had very little to offer to patients in such circumstances, and that for this patient to stand a chance, they would require far longer treatment, preferably in a specialized detox facility. Lindy next contacted a detox facility, one known for its successful treatment protocols, directly. After she presented the case and faxed all of the necessary clinical and insurance information, the intake personnel assured her that they could get the treatment approved and would handle prior authorization directly. After two days, we were informed by the detox facility that the insurance company needed more information. So, Lindy was back on the phone with them. Near five o'clock that day, Lindy was still on the phone, and her frustration was beginning to show. The insurance company employee on the other end of the line, already a supervisor of the first person Lindy had dealt with, claimed that it would take more time to get an accession number and nothing could be done to expedite this process. But the longer this process took, the more likely it was that our patient would go for their next fix.

I got on the phone next. I made it clear to this insurance company staffer that I was writing this book, and that if this process was not completed in the next thirty seconds, her name and the name of the insurance company would appear in this story. She placed me on hold and seconds later had the accession number for me. I was happy to have budged the process forward but angry to find that the company had clearly been stonewalling, despite the risk to the patient.

It still took two more days to make the arrangements for treatment to begin, but we were fortunate—no further harm befell our patient. The family was exceedingly grateful for our efforts but also told us a very disturbing story. They knew another family that was going through a similar situation at the same time. But their family member did not get the treatment they needed in time and did, in fact, overdose and die.

The Lie

In order to receive care in certain circumstances, someone may need to, shall we say, bend the truth. Now, let me just say up front, I would never do this, and my staff would never do such an abhorrent thing—bend the truth in order to save someone's life—because that would be fraud. But let's just say that we've heard of patients or other medical personnel who have behaved in such a terrible way. It goes without saying that we would rather let our patients forego food for expensive medications, go heavily into debt or even bankruptcy, or even die than commit fraud.

Here's an example of the Lie in action. A patient over the age of fifty was experiencing abdominal pain, a change in his bowel habits, and weight loss. These are symptoms that could be a sign of something as serious as colon cancer. An appropriate medical evaluation would include lab testing, a CT scan of the abdomen, and a colonoscopy. Unfortunately, the patient had a health insurance policy with a huge deductible and was not independently wealthy, so he could not afford to pay for all this in addition to the privilege of paying for his health insurance policy.

The labs and the CT scan were out of the question because of the cost. But the patient knew that his insurance was required to pay 100 percent for cancer-screening tests like a colonoscopy. All he had to do when he went to the doctor was lie and say that there was nothing wrong with him. That's what he did, and the colonoscopy was arranged.

Imagine the conversation between the patient and the doctor.

"What brings you in today?" asks the doctor.

"Oh, nothing," says the patient.

"Then why are you here?" the doctor asks.

Patient replies, "I just like to talk to you, Doc. Oh, and by the way, can you order me a colonoscopy?"

"Is something wrong?" the doctor asks.

"No, I just always wanted a colonoscopy, that's all."

The funny part is that patients tell us that, when they have their colonoscopies, if something significant like a polyp or tumor is found, then the colonoscopy is no longer considered a screening test, and the patient ends up having to pay for it. So, if my patient with the abdominal complaints actually has something wrong with him, like cancer, then he has to pay. Joke's on him, right?

Another version of the Lie is when someone who has a serious medical problem but can't afford insurance asks me to say they are disabled so they can qualify for Medicaid and then get what might be lifesaving care. That's right. An able-bodied person asks me to say they are disabled so they can get their medical care. Once again, that would be fraud. I would never commit fraud. Who cares if the patient dies? Fraud is wrong.

The Bargain

The Bargain is what takes place when patients with no insurance or high-deductible insurance negotiate how much they are willing to spend, weighing the cost against the potential seriousness of their medical condition. In other words, the more potentially serious the medical condition, the more most people are willing to spend. The Bargain is a new approach to medical care with many nuances. There are two basic Bargain strategies that patients employ: there is the low-spending Bargain and the high-spending Bargain.

The low-spending Bargain is when a patient has insurance with a huge deductible and they are trying to limit their medical care to the minimum amount because it comes out of their pocket. So, we bargain up to the value of their death. We try to minimize their medical expenses to the point that we think we might be missing a life-threatening condition, at which point we discuss how much a patient is willing to spend to avoid dying. This can get tricky, especially if a patient brings their spouse and they differ on how much the other is worth. For instance, if a patient has a hefty life insurance policy and we guess that evaluating and treating their condition is too expensive, the other spouse might opt for the life insurance instead.

A typical Bargain might go something like this. The patient mentioned in the previous section, who has abdominal pain, might ask if there isn't something we could do just to make it go away. That's a tough one, because without testing, it is hard to know just what is wrong. However, we can often try a medication, either an antacid or an antibiotic, empirically. I have to explain to the patient in such circumstances that if we don't obtain the testing, we might be missing some serious condition, risking things like death and all that. They're usually okay with that, at least at first.

113

I will typically bring that patient back after a month, and then we Bargain again. If their symptoms are all gone, then they Bargain to stop there. If they still have symptoms, then we Bargain for at least a first round of testing.

This is all well and good except that people do die this way. I had a patient a few years back whose Medicaid insurance policy did not cover expensive testing or specialist referrals. He developed abdominal pain. We did the Bargain and treated him for a time with medication. He didn't have a choice because he didn't have any money to obtain any further care. Finally, after about six months, we were able to figure out a Workaround and got him the testing that revealed his stomach cancer. He died about a year later.

The high-spending Bargain occurs when someone thinks there might be something seriously wrong with them and they want to get their money's worth from their insurance, which only kicks in after they have spent their deductible. They want you to order as much testing as you can so they hit their deductible as quickly as possible and then receive the benefit of their insurance. The tough part comes when this happens near the end of the year. People know that their deductible kicks back in on January 1, so if they develop a medical problem late in the year, they want you to get as much done as possible prior to the end of the year. This actually happens, and people beg you to do as much as possible so they don't face their high deductible twice. The implication is that you need to get sick early in the year so you can get the full value of your health insurance. I wouldn't be surprised to see statistics that show that claims rise late in the year and fall early in the year because of this.

Another form of the Bargain is when patients wait until their insurance kicks in to receive care. I had one uninsured patient opt to wait more than a year, until their Medicare kicked in, to seek treatment for a serious cancer. I had another who endured a heart attack at home and waited more than a year to seek cardiac care when their Medicare coverage began.

You Better Find Something Wrong with Me

Things get really interesting for people who have high-deductible health insurance once they have gotten to the point in the Bargain where they are afraid something could be seriously wrong with them. Out of concern for their health and safety, they decide to spend whatever it takes. Sometimes, though, they spend all that money only to find that nothing is wrong. They can get pretty angry if you waste their deductible and don't find out that they have cancer or something nasty like that. So, you have to hope that if you go to the trouble of spending their deductible, at least they have cancer. I am not making this up—people have gotten angry with me because they don't have cancer.

The Fix

If I have one piece of advice that would be of most value, it is "Don't get sick." I'm serious. The last thing you want is to need this medical system because it may harm you as much as it may help. So, get your exercise, eat a healthy diet, try to control your weight, and do not smoke. That is your best insurance policy by far.

On a bigger scale, what is needed is affordable *universal care* rather than a system that is trying unsuccessfully to achieve *universal insurance*. Universal care means everyone is in the system—100 percent of the population is included, and everyone has access to necessary care. Universal care also means that all reasonable medical care is covered. What is reasonable would be determined by national consensus. And what is deemed reasonable could be obtained with an order from a physician or other health-care professional. There would be no authorization processes or incomplete coverage for such care.

This brings us to the political side of the issue. How can we deliver and pay for a universal care model? The most obvious way is through a single-payer system. A single-payer system would bring simplicity and clarity to an American health-care system that badly needs it. But before you get your anti-socialist hackles up, I will say that single payer is not the only way we could achieve universal care, just the simplest. An insurance-based system could deliver the same thing, but universal care with everybody in and 100 percent coverage of reasonable care would have to be legislated into the system. We could achieve the same by instituting a public option insurance policy as previously discussed, as well.

Affordability is central to an improved health-care system. Affordability requires that everyone has access at a reasonable cost and a reasonable cap on out-of-pocket expenses. Numbers that have been discussed in such a system, and seem appropriate, would be 4 to 5 percent of income, with a maximum of $5,000–$7,500 total cost per year. In an insurance-based system, government could subsidize premiums above that amount. Substantial co-pays and deductibles are just a bad idea for patients, and they should be eliminated altogether. If patients and their doctors feel they need care, they should receive it!

CHAPTER 6

Measuring the Quality of Medical Care Is Bad for You

Mary is a seventy-five-year-old patient with a history of diabetes, high blood pressure, and migraine headaches who comes in for a regular checkup. I've known Mary for years, and we've been through a lot together over the years. I also take care of Mary's husband, daughter, and grandchild. Mary is feeling well today.

She takes the medications metformin and Januvia for her diabetes. I normally try to avoid brand-name medications like Januvia because of their expense, but Mary has an allergy to sulfa drugs, which prevents me from prescribing less expensive and more commonly used diabetes medications called the sulfonylureas, which derive from the sulfa medication family. In fact, Mary shows me a letter she recently received from her pharmacy benefits administrator stating that the amount she will have to pay for the Januvia will soon be going up substantially and encouraging her to ask me to prescribe a different medication, if possible.

We review Mary's labs. Her hemoglobin A1c (HgbA1c), the test used most often to measure diabetes control, has slowly been rising. At her most recent visit six months ago, the HgbA1c was 7.2. This time, it has gone up to 7.8. Our goal is to try to keep the HgbA1c as close to 7 as possible. In fact, for many years, well-known guidelines for the care of diabetes published by the American Diabetes Association (ADA) had recommended that the HgbA1c should be kept below 7. However, more recent studies have suggested that keeping the value of the HgbA1c under 8, and maybe even 9, may achieve many of the same benefits. Recent studies have also shown that very low HgbA1c levels, near 6 or lower, actually result in poorer outcomes. Therefore, the ADA recently revised its recommendations, suggesting that patients and their doctors individualize the goals for HgbA1c in each patient.

Mary's cholesterol is high. The ADA and the American Heart Association both recommend that people with diabetes be treated with the well-known cholesterol-lowering medications, the statins, because they have been shown to lower the risks of cardiac disease in diabetics so substantially. Unfortunately, Mary has attempted to take four different statin medications but experienced intense muscle soreness, a well-known side effect, with each one. We have even considered trying a fifth statin, but Mary's Medicare D prescription plan does not cover any of the remaining drugs in this class, and she cannot afford to pay the exorbitant price for the non-covered drugs. So, Mary is not on a statin.

Mary's blood pressure this visit is 144/88. In the past, the recommended goal for blood pressure in a diabetic was less than 130/80. More recently, though, it was recognized that keeping the blood pressure this low might not offer the benefits we once thought it did and may even lead to harm in certain circumstances. Mary takes Lisinopril, a type of blood pressure medication that is strongly recommended for people who have diabetes because it has been shown to protect kidney function. She had been on a higher dose of Lisinopril previously but had complained of feeling weak and dizzy. We both feared that dizziness could lead to a fall, and we therefore decided to stick with the current dose of Lisinopril even if the blood pressure was a tiny bit higher than we would have liked.

Mary also had a long history of migraine headaches. Prior to treatment of her headaches, Mary would have a severely disabling migraine almost once per week. Thankfully, we had found a medication that was controlling her headaches very well. Mary was taking amitriptyline, a medication commonly used for this purpose. Amitriptyline can cause significant side effects in some patients, primarily drowsiness, but many people can take the medication without any problems. Mary has been on amitriptyline for years. Every time she has a checkup, we review how she is doing with this medication and whether she is having any side effects. She continues to do well.

So, everything is going well except that I just received a quality report card from Mary's Medicare administrator. The report noted that Mary's HgbA1c have been over 7 and that her systolic (the higher number) blood pressures have been over 140. They also note that Mary is not on a statin medication, and that amitriptyline is on a list of medications known as the Beers Criteria, which identifies potentially inappropriate medications for older adults.

I would normally have ignored such quality report cards, but more and more, the data in reports such as this one is being used to rate physicians and health systems; it forms the basis of financial incentives and penalties. For instance, recent federal regulations have created a new payment model known as the Accountable Care Organization (ACO) that brings together large numbers of physicians who are paid based on their performance on a huge set of quality metrics. In addition to requiring that doctors join such ACOs, CMS has announced that a significant portion of a physician's pay, starting in the year 2019, is going to be based on their quality metric performance (this program is discussed in detail in Chapter 8).

Mary is a pretty typical patient in my practice. As with the multitude of other patients like her, we have worked together to find a reasonable balance of a complex mixture that includes satisfying clinical guidelines, working within monetary and insurance-related constraints, and avoiding potential medication side effects to hammer out a commonsense strategy to care for her numerous chronic medical conditions. And, as I said, Mary is doing well. However, the growing reliance on quality metrics as a basis for physician pay, known alternatively as "pay for performance" or "value-based pay," rather than improving my care, actually inhibits best care in many circumstances and even encourages bad care.

It Looks Good on Paper

Nowhere is the bureaucracy more at odds with common sense and the reality of clinical medicine than when it comes to the topic of quality metrics. Quality metrics are the bureaucracy's declaration of war on doctors. Tying payments to performance data is their weapon of mass destruction.

The concepts underlying "value-based pay" would seem to make sense and would not be entirely without merit if used in a balanced and reasonable manner. But balance and reason are in short supply these days at CMS.

There is a multitude of well-known and well-researched standards that help guide and define optimal clinical care. These include numerical targets for things like blood pressure, cholesterol, and blood sugar control in diabetes; standards for preventive care, such as cancer screenings and immunizations; and guidelines that recommend the most effective and appropriate medications to use for various diagnoses and clinical scenarios. Too often, though, many of these standards of care go unmet. It is a significant problem that results in suboptimal patient outcomes, and suboptimal patient outcomes then lead to unnecessary medical expenditures. And this goes directly to the heart of what is wrong with the low-quality, high-cost American health-care system.

There are various schools of thought regarding quality improvement, and the use of objective data to guide decision-making is key to many of those approaches. Accordingly, it seems fit that one of the ways to improve American health care would be to measure doctors' performance on known standards of care and then to base payment on the results—this forms the basis of pay-for-performance (P4P) or value-based payment models. It has become traditional to both offer incentives when standards are met and to use penalties if they are not.

But as the above clinical vignette demonstrates, things may not be as cut and dry as they seem. What seems black and white to the untrained clinical eye, may, in the complex world of health care, have many shades of gray. Rather than improve quality and reduce the costs of care, value-based pay, as it is currently being used, results in unintended consequences that undermine that intent. This chapter shines a light on these issues and suggests a more effective way forward.

Managing Costs through Performance Improvement

The twin plagues of low quality and high cost were the basis of criticisms leveled at the American medical system even as Bill and Hillary Clinton took on health-care reform in the early 1990s. When their efforts failed, policy-makers turned to managed care models that used capitated payments (fixed, pre-arranged payments that covered a period of time, usually a month) rather than traditional fee-for-service payments (where physicians are paid for each service, such as an appointment or a particular procedure) in an effort to control costs. With no emphasis on controlling the quality of care, however, capitated models resulted chiefly in less care (the less care and the fewer tests or treatments a patient received, the more money the physician or hospital made), but less care was not better care, and by the end of the 1990s, the managed care fad had gone out of style along with grunge rock.

The lesson policy-makers came away with from this experience was that there must be an emphasis placed on both performance improvement *and* lower costs. In fact, many felt that higher-quality medical care, in and of itself, would inevitably lead to lower cost, and a P4P strategy was the key. Many of these programs began to spring up in the private sector in the early 2000s.

In 2005, the federally funded community clinic where I practiced and at which I was the medical director began participating in one such performance-improvement project, referred to as a "disease collaborative," which was a program intended to improve care, and therefore lower expenditures, for important (and costly) chronic medical conditions such as diabetes and heart disease. We enrolled in a diabetes collaborative.

The primary emphasis of the program, at least initially, was collecting data—lots of data. It was felt that in order to improve performance and even just to discuss clinical quality, there needed to be data that would serve as a reference point at the outset of the project and then periodically as a metric for gauging the progress of any performance-improvement efforts. What we would do with that data—how we would use the data to improve performance— was less clear.

At mandatory meetings attended by all of the participating community clinics in our region, we were encouraged to return to our clinics and perform rapid cycles of quality-improvement PDSA (plan-do-study-act) projects, a popular performance-improvement technique, in the hopes that we would come up with ways (the program leaders didn't seem to know many) to improve care, and hence our data, as well.

But the first order of business was data collection, which turned out to be easier said than done. There was a great deal of both demographic and clinical data (i.e., diagnoses, medications, and the results of blood pressure measurements, to name just a few) required by the program. And at that time, almost all this data was hidden inside patients' paper charts. So, we began the imposing task of compiling data from every chart of every diabetic patient in our practice. We would record the data for each chart on paper forms and then input the data into specialized computer registries.

Almost immediately two problems became apparent. First and foremost, the reality was that it took so much time and effort to compile and report the data that we could do little else. The immense energy it took to collect all of this data supplanted almost all efforts to improve the care that was reflected in the data. In fact, ongoing data collection proved so time-consuming that we actually had to hire extra staff to complete it. This meant additional costs, of course (though we hired high school students, who worked for cheap but I doubt did the best work).

Second, even with extra staff, it took so long to extract and report our data that by the time any meaningful results were available, so much time had elapsed that the data was no longer of any particular use. By the time the patient was back in our office, the data was often out of date.

And, all the while, this huge effort did little to encourage improved clinical care. So, the end result of our new program was a great deal of extra effort, additional costs, and no improvement in performance. It was apparent that collecting data did not necessarily result in improved performance, and that this approach, so central to P4P, might not be all it was cracked up to be.

P4P in the Computer Era

For obvious reasons, P4P in the era of paper charting was extraordinarily challenging. Certainly, one of the great promises of health information technology is the ability to cull data much more easily and on a much larger scale than was previously possible. But in reality, not all computer systems are created equal, and consequently, not all systems can collect or spit out data equally.

On top of that, in addition to documenting traditional aspects of medical care, medical professionals now must also document compliance with numerous performance-improvement metrics. The extra time and focus can be considerable.

In July 2015, the American Medical Association hosted a town hall meeting as part of their Break the Red Tape initiative, where physicians were encouraged to share their experiences with EHRs. Gary Botstein, MD, a Dekatur, Georgia, rheumatologist reported, "In my program I have to collect large amounts of data. . . . Once all this data was collected you couldn't even find it. As opposed to looking at the patient, thinking about what's important with this patient, asking the relevant questions, then proceeding to take care of this patient, there's this huge fountain of collection of data, then you've got to go wading through it hoping you can find the relevant piece of information. It's a totally backwards approach."

At the same meeting, V. K. Puppula, MD, a pain medicine specialist, commented, "We're basically being turned into data miners in order to spend all of our time and effort on documentation as opposed to the key issue of medical decision-making."

There is a growing list of mandatory performance-improvement initiatives, each with its own set of uniquely defined clinical quality metrics. The vast amount of data being collected has very important implications for both data quality and our ability to put that data to any use. Quite simply, more is less in this case. The huge and growing bureaucratic obsession with data once again defeats its own purpose.

This is just a sampling of the various performance-improvement programs physicians may be required to participate in:

1. Meaningful Use (MU): nine clinical quality measures
2. Physician Quality Reporting System (PQRS): nine clinical quality measures
3. Patient Centered Medical Homes (PCMH): eight clinical quality measures
4. Accountable Care Organizations (ACO): thirty-three clinical quality measures

I can assure you it has become too much. The cult of data has taken over. We spend so much time trying to keep abreast of the changes associated with each of these programs, and then documenting compliance with every new measure, that it is all we can do. So once again, just like when my community clinic attempted P4P in the paper era, there is no time left to improve performance. The data is an end unto itself.

The push to reduce every aspect of medical care to a number has other negative implications. When these vast quantities of data are tied to money—the incentives, but especially the penalties of P4P—and hence the pressure to demonstrate certain results mounts, it has implications for the accuracy of the data and even provides the impetus to commit fraud.

For instance, I have heard, anecdotally, of a health system that massages its data in order to achieve the necessary thresholds to earn Medicare's new post-hospitalization follow-up incentives. In 2014, in an effort to reduce the rate of readmissions following a hospital stay, Medicare began to offer special payments for patients who are seen again within seven to fourteen days of discharge. This represents big money to a health system that can demonstrate compliance. Medicare also maintains a consumer website called Hospital Compare that provides information on a hospital's performance on such measures. One doctor told me that his health system regularly reviews their data and then removes patients from their calculation's denominator (the number of patients that are discharged from the hospital and require follow-up appointments) to improve the appearance of their results. Unfortunately, this type of behavior becomes almost inevitable when the pressures and monetary implications are so great.

So, from these experiences, we learn a very important lesson about data-driven performance improvement: while data is an important aspect of performance improvement, collecting it in a way that requires an inordinate amount of time and work can destroy such efforts. And there is a logical corollary to this: focusing on a few achievable data-driven performance objectives is better than collecting massive amounts of data with no specific plan to improve performance. In other words, less is often more.

Medicine by the Numbers

Conceptually, P4P is problematic in a host of other ways that make its appropriateness and applicability questionable and its conflicts with the realities of medical care apparent.

The number one problem is that metrics reduce patient care to simplistic scenarios that just do not match the complexity encountered in the real world. While standards of care are useful in helping to guide medical decision-making, there are frequent instances when strict adherence to a numeric goal or simple clinical rule is inappropriate, encourages bad care, and may even discourage clinicians from caring for certain patient populations.

As the clinical vignette at the beginning of this chapter demonstrates, there are times when it is in the patient's best interest that their blood pressure be a little higher than what is usual. Many older patients suffer from bouts of dizziness or unsteadiness, and a lower blood pressure might worsen their symptoms, and increase their risks of falling, or make them less willing to be active. Similarly, some patients have a tendency toward dangerously low blood sugars and may be better off if their blood sugar is allowed to remain slightly higher than what is desirable for other patients.

And when it comes to treating pain and even many psychiatric conditions in older individuals, it is often necessary and appropriate to use medications that are deemed inappropriate by the Beers Criteria (mentioned previously). These medications are often very effective, and when used with appropriate caution and monitoring, can be very safe. Without these options, we would lose what is often our best method for dealing with older patients' very real pain and emotional suffering.

The best medical care is individualized and nuanced, and it is best determined by the clinical team working closely with the patient, not by a bean counter applying rules that cannot distinguish between what is clinically right and wrong. Metrics are the mandatory sentencing guidelines of medicine.

Overreliance on metrics (as opposed to common sense) also penalizes physicians who see the most challenging patient populations. Older patients, who tend to carry more serious diagnoses and pose unique clinical and social challenges, naturally generate worse clinical data even when they receive exquisitely good care. Rural patients, poor patients, patients with serious chronic conditions, and certain ethnic populations pose similar challenges. Under P4P programs, doctors who care for these special patient populations will be penalized! This is exactly the opposite of what we want.

The size of a clinician's particular patient population also affects their data. In my community clinic, we regularly analyzed data for our diabetic patients. Every month, we would run reports for each of the clinician's HgbA1c results. I saw far more diabetic patients than anyone else in the practice, and surprisingly, my HgbA1c average tended to be the lowest. I would like to think that my low numbers reflected the excellent quality of my care, but the fact is that having higher numbers of patients also smoothed out any abnormally high HgbA1c results my patients may have had. For the other clinicians, lower patient numbers meant that any high HgbA1c reading had a much larger effect on their averages. Hence, without adjusting for the number of patients being seen, it would be inappropriate to make too much out of the differences noted in our results. So, once again, P4P may not actually be able to distinguish good care from bad and may penalize physicians inappropriately.

The American Health-Care System Destroys Quality

The financial barriers and the barriers to medical care created by the uninsured and underinsured patients that define American health care often prevent doctors from practicing optimal care. Insurance policies with high deductibles, difficult prior authorization processes for testing and medications, and restrictive prescription formularies cause the same problem. It is a cruel joke to pressure doctors to achieve performance standards and then systematically prevent their achieving them. And yet, this is exactly what we do. It's like we're entered into hell's egg-tossing contest and our hands are tied behind our backs.

One of the cruelest of the jokes is that insulin, the lifeblood of the clinical care of many diabetic patients, is becoming increasingly expensive. Elderly patients now regularly report to me that their insulins can cost hundreds of dollars per prescription. And often, the convenient pen syringes that make insulin injection much safer and simpler for those patients are not covered and are priced out of patients' reach. And each new diabetes medication released by the pharmaceutical industry is priced out of reach, as well—the approximate retail price of Tradjenta is listed at $410 for a thirty-day supply; the popular inject-able medication Victoza is $1,500 per month; Invokana is $450 for a month's supply. It is obscene, and it makes caring for patients with dia-betes exceedingly difficult if not impossible. And yet, we are expected to hit the marks on diabetes care or incur a penalty.

Satisfied Patients Get More Pain Medications and Antibiotics

One of the newer "quality domains," as defined by CMS, is the "Patient-Caregiver Experience," sometimes also referred to as "patient engagement," which is just a fancy term for patient satisfac-tion surveys. A portion of a hospital's pay is now dependent on the results of surveys performed as part of the Consumer Assessment of Healthcare Providers and Systems (CAHPS) program. Over the coming years, these same types of assessments will be required for outpatient practices as part of expanding P4P programs, as well.

Not only does this represent one more addition to the already burgeoning pile of questionable administrative requirements, it also requires providers to hire vendors to perform such surveys. The dreaded Press Ganey survey (Press Ganey is the company that per-forms most hospital patient satisfaction surveys and has a virtual monopoly on this market) is much maligned for both its techniques and its questionable results. Far worse, however, is what is done to those whose scores don't make the grade. Demeaning meetings with administrators and rehabilitation are becoming common.

A January 2013 article in *Forbes* titled "Why Rating Your Doctor is Bad for Your Health" describes many of the negative aspects of the Press Ganey mentality: "The little-known company has become a hated target of hospital physicians, outstripping even trial lawyers. Utter its name in an emergency room and you'll likely unleash a cloud of four-letter words. . . . Many doctors, in order to get high ratings (and a higher salary), overprescribe and overtest, just to 'satisfy' patients, who probably aren't qualified to judge their care. And there's a financial cost, as flawed survey methods and the decisions they induce, produce billions more in waste. It's a case of good intentions gone badly awry—and it's only getting worse." Sound familiar?

The inevitable result of this misguided bureaucratic stupidity is that physicians will do whatever it takes to make patients happy, which is often not in the patient's or society's best interest, like over-prescribing narcotics or antibiotics, or going easy on noncompliant patients, who might just benefit from a swift kick from time to time. The *Forbes* article makes this clear: "One emergency room with poor survey scores started offering Vicodin 'goody bags' to discharged patients in order to improve their ratings. And doctors face the reality that uncomfortable discussions on behavioral topics—say, smoking or obesity—come with the risk of a pay cut."

It is obvious to everyone except the government bureaucrats who impose these idiotic demands that patients are not customers. So, while customers may always be right, patients are not, and this is just not an appropriate way to view patient care. Doctors and nurses are not waitresses, maître d's, concierges, or salespeople, and they should not be rated in the same way.

Of course, we want patients to be respected, well treated, and involved in their care as much as is possible and desirable. We want them to be and to feel well cared for. It is a profoundly important aspect of the best patient care, but patient satisfaction surveys are not the way to accomplish this and may in many ways encourage the opposite.

Financial Penalties Destroy the Doctor-Patient Relationship—Thanks, Obama

Satisfaction surveys create incentives for physicians to provide inappropriate care to patients, but financial penalties have the potential to just outright destroy the doctor-patient relationship. If I am going to be penalized, and lose income, because my patients' numbers do not pass muster, then I just might not want to take care of patients with challenging issues.

In the past, my staff and I tended to view many of the patients with the most challenging medical, social, and mental health issues as the ones we relished taking care of the most, because we took satisfaction in overcoming the obstacles they presented. Maybe we are clinical gluttons for punishment in this way, but in fact, we love it. We take satisfaction in helping the people who need it the most.

But if we are going to be penalized monetarily for taking care of these patients, and on top of that, have to deal with the systematic barriers that prevent us from giving them good care, then they are no longer desirable patients. Worse still, sometimes these patients don't do what we ask, don't listen to us, don't take care of themselves, or even seem interested in such things. Being penalized under such circumstances encourages an adversarial situation—the furthest thing from what is desirable or helpful when it comes to taking care of patients!

But the situation will be even worse because of the particularly harmful way that CMS has designed its new P4P system, set to begin in 2019. As it is currently planned, 50 percent of doctors will be penalized in this system no matter what level of care they provide and regardless of the results of their quality scorecard. CMS will identify a median performance level among all physicians (this rating scale is discussed in detail in Chapter 8), and whoever is below the median will receive a penalty, while whoever is above the median will get an incentive payment. So, it is possible that a physician could have reasonably good clinical quality scores and still receive a reduction in pay. I would love to see bureaucrats and administrators (you could throw in politicians, as well) have their salaries tied to their performance in such ways.

For all of these reasons, using clinical quality measures or satisfaction surveys to penalize doctors and health systems is a bad idea that, maybe more than any other issue, highlights what goes wrong when bureaucrats and administrators have too much control while patients and their clinical teams have too little. I get angry just thinking about it, and so should you.

Does P4P Work?

I think I have made a very clear and compelling case against over-reliance on clinical quality data. And the reality is that these models have been tried and tested, and the results are not impressive. The notion so beloved in bureaucratic circles that measuring data, and tying that data to monetary incentives and penalties, magically leads to improved results is not supported by real-world experiences.

A May 30, 2015, review of the P4P experience in *Modern Healthcare* titled "Physician Quality Pay Not Paying Off" argues, "While offering physicians bonuses for hitting quality benchmarks is popular, the incentive programs may not be worth the money. Linking financial rewards to cost-effective management of patient care or reducing adverse outcomes has not produced the desired results, recent studies show. When it comes to physician pay, some experts are asking if healthcare organizations are moving in the wrong direction."

The review also quotes Dr. Steffie Woolhandler, a professor at the City University of New York's School of Public Health: "There is essentially no evidence that pay-for-performance works, and certainly no evidence that it works as it is being applied to American health care right now."

An October 2012 article in *Health Affairs*, "Pay for Performance," included a review of numerous such projects, and the results were not encouraging: "Andrew M. Ryan at Cornell University and colleagues studied the first years of the Massachusetts Medicaid hospital pay-for-performance program, which offered financial incentives for improving care for pneumonia and prevention of surgical infections, and found no improvement in quality. Another study led by Steven D. Pearson of Massachusetts General Hospital compared quality performance among Massachusetts' physician group practices during 2001–03 and found improvement in quality measures across all of the medical groups, regardless of whether or not pay-for-performance incentives were in place."

So, P4P models have not been shown to be particularly effective. Despite that fact, and all of P4P's potential for harmful consequences, bureaucrats have made it the centerpiece of their efforts to reform health-care delivery and payments to physicians and health systems in the United States. It boggles the mind and upsets my digestive tract!

Data Is Just One Aspect of Performance Improvement

The issues highlighted by these research results, and by the preceding critique of P4P, are that clinical quality is more than simple metrics and that improved performance is not the inevitable outcome of measuring data and tying it to financial carrots and sticks.

What I think is clear is that measuring data is just one small aspect of performance improvement. My clinic's experiences in the previously mentioned diabetes collaborative were illustrative of that fact, as was our approach after this became clear.

With great fanfare, we had announced to the staff our plans to improve the quality of our care, had offered incentives and awards, and periodically measured the specified clinical metrics. After a few rounds of measuring and reporting the data, we recognized that all we were accomplishing was—measuring and reporting data. The results didn't change. We soon recognized the pointlessness of this effort, but also learned a very important lesson. We were missing an integral step. If we wanted performance to improve, we needed to specifically address how that would happen.

From a medicine perspective, there are four aspects of diabetes care that must be addressed with every patient:

1. Controlling blood sugars (rated by a patient's HgbA1c result)
2. Use of daily aspirin
3. Use of a type of blood pressure medication knows as an ACE inhibitor
4. Use of the statin cholesterol medications

Controlling blood sugar can be very difficult and is often quite complicated, so we avoided that aspect in our project. The other three items on the list are simple to address. A quick and straightforward analysis can determine whether a patient should or shouldn't use an aspirin, an ACE inhibitor, and a statin. And improvements in patient outcomes related to use of these three types of medications in diabetic patients are substantial.

From our data collection efforts, we had baseline information on the percentages of diabetic patients in our practice who were using these three medications. We pulled the charts of every diabetic patient in our practice not using each of the three medications. The charts were then distributed to the patients' primary clinician who then had the opportunity to add medications as appropriate.

Then, we measured the data again. The numbers of patients who were now using all three medications went up dramatically! With this one project, we improved our data, but more importantly, significantly improved patient care.

So, data is most useful when it is being used as part of a comprehensive performance-improvement effort. Unfortunately, this is not what CMS has planned.

The Fix

This is so simple. It is not that we shouldn't be measuring and using clinical quality data, it's that we need to be doing it right.

Rule number one is that less is more. You might as well just throw in the "keep it simple, stupid" (KISS) rule. They almost always go together. The emphasis should be on a very limited number of measures; results on those measures should be exceedingly easy to record and report (this entire process should be as automated as possible, if not entirely automated); and each measure must be part of a comprehensive plan to improve performance. I would suggest that each medical specialty work on two or three measures per year as part of a fully planned national ten-year performance-improvement initiative.

Priority should be given to simple evidence-based interventions that are easy and inexpensive to implement and that have known substantial and predictable impacts. An example of such a measure is use of the statin cholesterol medications in the setting of coronary artery disease. This is simple from almost every angle, and the results are automatically recorded when a clinician records a diagnosis and the use of the appropriate medication, both of which are documented while performing typical aspects of clinical care.

Measures that should be avoided are ones that may be difficult to implement and satisfy, that take extra effort to record, or that have unproven or difficult to quantify impacts. A good example of a measure to avoid in P4P initiatives would be lifestyle counseling for overweight patients. I believe there is value in lifestyle counseling, and it is something that I do with many of my patients, but it is a poorly defined concept that takes extra effort to record and has unclear benefits.

Rule number two is that there should be no penalties tied to performance improvement as it pertains to patient care. The unintended consequences are just too great.

Third, all barriers to care that relate to a measure must be removed. For instance, if we are going to measure performance related to childhood and adult immunizations, which is a good idea, we should also identify alternative models to better deliver this important service. This could include increased utilization of health departments, or even better, distributing immunizations at no cost to physician practices, who often avoid giving immunizations because of the huge and growing upfront outlays to purchase inventory in conjunction with often disappointing reimbursements. In addition, all reasonable care that relates to any measure selected should be mandated to be fully covered by insurance.

And finally, we should also define specific ways to leverage technology and other resources to assist clinicians in achieving clinical goals. Rather than using penalties, we should be identifying ways that we can make clinical care easier and more effective. For instance, in those very rare circumstances where one of my diabetic patients, especially those on complicated insulin regimens, could use more help than I can easily provide, it would be outstanding, and much appreciated, if I had a reliable and readily available service where I could refer such patients. As it stands, I do not.

In fact, it would be amazing to think that I worked within a system that actually helped me take better care of my patients rather than the current one that tries to trip me up and then takes money from me when I actually fall down. We can at least imagine.

CHAPTER 7

Patient-Centered Medical Homes— How to Make a Simple Solution Unattainable

Many people by now have heard of the new practice management concept that is sweeping the nation—the patient-centered medical home, better known by its abbreviation, PCMH. PCMHs are touted as the latest and greatest fix to our ailing health-care system. PCMH models are being adopted all over the nation, and "patient-centeredness" has become a recognized phrase in medical terminology. It has taken on an almost cultlike status. PCMHs are so highly regarded by the Centers for Medicare and Medicaid Services that the organization has deemed participation in a specialized form of the model one of the ways that a physician can satisfy the requirements of the transition to a value-based payment system that begins in 2019. Very few in the medical community seem to question any of this. I am, apparently, a heretic in this respect.

What is a PCMH? As the National Committee for Quality Assurance (NCQA), the organization that has probably done the most to define the PCMH model, describes it, "patient-centered medical homes (PCMH) transform primary care practices into what patients want: health care that focuses on them and their needs. PCMHs get to know patients in long-term partnerships, rather than through hurried, sporadic visits. They make treatment decisions with their patients, based on patient preference. They help patients become engaged in their own healthy behaviors and health care."

Under this model, "everyone in the practice—from clinicians to front desk staff—works as a team to coordinate care with other providers and community resources. This maximizes efficiency by ensuring that highly trained clinicians are not performing tasks that can be accomplished by other staff, and helps avoid costly and preventable complications and emergencies through a focus on prevention and managing chronic conditions."

Sounds great, doesn't it? And conceptually, in many ways, it is. But in its everything-but-the-kitchen-sink reality, it becomes just another example of more—more rules, more fads, and more documentation and data collection—being less.

Why Do We Need PCMHs?

Most of the concepts underlying the PCMH model are not new. Maybe you will find this hard to believe, but doctors in training are taught to provide comprehensive, accessible, holistic care. In my first year of medical school, in an era long ago (1993), I was introduced to the biopsychosocial model of patient care, which taught that patients were more than just a collection of their strictly medical symptoms and treatments. The model teaches the broad view that patient problems should be considered in the context of various biological, psychological, and social factors. We were also taught that optimal patient care was more than just episodic disease diagnoses and treatment—that the best care also included chronic disease management: systematic management of preventive health, such as immunizations and cancer screenings; and shared decision-making, with a hefty dose of patient education, all within the context of a long-term relationship between a patient and his or her medical team. And then later, during my family medicine residency (1997–2000, when my hair began to turn prematurely gray), we were taught that part of our task was to serve as the hub of a patient's medical experience—that we were to guide and coordinate our patients' care through the medical system if and when they required hospital or specialist treatments.

Apparently, somewhere between our training and the eventual realities of practicing medicine, something goes awry, because many doctors and their practices then ignore these crucial aspects of patient care. The financial bottom line and the extra burdens created by a dysfunctional health-care system—well documented in previous chapters—take over, and medical care degenerates into a rush of disjointed episodic appointments with physicians who are pushed to see more patients at an ever-faster pace.

Whereas in residency we trained to see patients in fifteen-minute time slots, already a significant challenge, once in practice, for many that may be reduced to five minutes or less. When that happens, something has to give, and that is usually high-quality comprehensive care. No one likes it. Patients, often after long waits, are rushed through their appointments. Doctors are frazzled and burned out.

The most popular medical practice management models (usually taught by non-physician consultants) contribute to the problem. The typical business model that physicians are taught focuses almost entirely on ways to increase patient volume—that seeing more patients generates more revenue and higher revenue is the overriding goal. This appears to make sense, of course, because doctors are paid primarily on a fee-for-service basis. And the most common application of this thinking is an efficiency model that teaches that doctors can see the most patients when they provide only those services that no one else can perform. They are taught to practice to the "highest level of their training," meaning that any task that might be done by someone other than a physician (in other words, less expensive staff) should be jettisoned to support staff. This way of thinking encourages physicians to hire as many support staff as might be necessary so that they can sprint from room to room maximizing their revenue.

And the lesson is further hammered home by administrators who judge a physician's worth according to productivity ratings such as the relative value unit (RVU). These calculations typically estimate physician productivity based on numbers of patients seen combined with average revenues per appointment. Many practices report physician RVUs on a regular basis and even tie salary and bonuses to the results. There is constant pressure to see more patients as a consequence.

But this business/efficiency model is problematic. The obvious result is an emphasis on patient volume over everything else. But the model is also based on a number of flawed assumptions. First of all, having physicians practicing to the "highest level of their training" is a nebulous concept. It is often taken to mean that physicians shouldn't waste their valuable time doing things like patient education, lifestyle coaching, or monitoring things like a patient's immunization or cancer screening status. But unloading a physician's responsibilities onto non-physicians does not necessarily result in better care, or even more efficient care, and financial limitations may limit a practice's ability to do such things anyway. In many instances, the physician may actually be the best person to handle those tasks. A physician's training, as well as their often unique standing in patients' lives, can give them an advantage in many circumstances.

Less obvious, but just as important, is the harmful effect of having to hire more and more support staff. The number one expense in most medical practices, by a long shot, is staff salaries. The average primary care office employs between three and seven staff per full-time clinician. The problem is that hiring more staff results in increased overhead expenses that can outstrip the extra revenue generated by seeing more patients. In other words, this model perpetuates the need to see ever higher numbers of patients. It is inherently flawed. It leads to lousy care and clinician burnout. And yet, it is the dominant thinking in medical practice management.

So the combination of a dysfunctional health-care system and an unhealthy practice environment, caused by common—but often mistaken—business practices, force physicians onto a hamster wheel of ever-increasing patient numbers. Comprehensive care goes by the wayside.

PCMH to the Rescue?

Into this void leapt the PCMH, which took shape as a formal model in the early 2000s. The NCQA first defined its version of the PCMH in 2007 in its "Joint Principles of the Patient-Centered Medical Home." Conceptually, the PCMH model attempts to create the type of care environment that all doctors were taught but are too often unable to deliver.

The PCMH prescription contains many good ideas, but the model, as it is most often defined, just goes way overboard. It mandates an overly long and detailed list of fixes, many of questionable value, and each tied to some documentation and data measurement requirement. It can increase administrative costs and staffing needs, further driving up a practice's overhead costs, creating the need to see even more patients, which undermines its purpose. The devil, as we have said over and over, is in the details.

As mentioned previously, one of the most widely accepted definitions of the PCMH comes from the National Committee for Quality Assurance. The NCQA has written extraordinarily detailed PCMH standards and guidelines and also functions as a certifying agency for official PCMH recognition. For the necessary detail to understand and to critique PCMH concepts, therefore, these guidelines are a good place to focus our attention.

According to the NCQA, "medical homes are the foundation for a health-care system that achieves the 'Triple Aim' of better quality, experience and cost." The NCQA describes its "Goals for PCMH and Beyond":

1. Primary care clinicians will deliver safe, effective and efficient care that is coordinated across the medical neighborhood and optimizes the patient experience.
2. Primary care will be the foundation of a high-value health-care system that provides whole-person care at the first contact. Everyone in primary care practices—from physicians and advanced practice nurses to medical assistants and front-line staff—should practice to the highest level of their training and license in teams, to support better access, self-care and care coordination.
3. PCMHs will show the entire health-care system what patient-centered care looks like: care that is "respectful of and responsive to individual patient preferences, needs, and values, and ensures that patient values guide all clinical decisions." Individuals and families get help to be actively engaged in their own healthy behaviors and health care, and in decisions about their care.

4. PCMHs will revitalize the "joy of practice" in primary care, making it more appealing and satisfying.

To be recognized as a PCMH, a practice or organization must be certified by the NCQA according to six detailed standards that cover:

1. Patient-Centered Access
2. Team-Based Care
3. Population Health Management
4. Care Management and Support
5. Care Coordination and Care Transitions
6. Performance Measurement and Quality Improvement

Getting on the Bandwagon

I should note that in 2011, my small practice became certified as a Level 2 (there are three levels of recognition) NCQA PCMH and began participation in a state-based PCMH pilot program. These experiences help form the basis of my critique.

Why did we choose to participate? Not surprisingly, money was the number one reason. Participation was tied to a payment of approximately $4 to $6 per participating patient per month. We were also to receive a share of any savings that the program generated, based on certain nebulous calculations. My practice had been founded on the concepts of accessible and comprehensive care. But much of our work of coordinating care and scheduling testing and specialty appointments went uncompensated. We reasoned— as many of the other participating practices did—that this was an opportunity to be paid for work we were already doing.

In order to participate in the pilot program, our practice needed to be NCQA certified by a certain date. My staff and I worked long hours to prepare the array of reports and data the program required. We submitted our completed application feeling confident. A number of months passed. But shortly before the pilot program's compliance deadline, we received word that we had, in fact, failed!

We contacted our NCQA auditor to find out what had gone wrong. The auditor was very busy, and the earliest she could meet with us was some days later at 7:30 in the evening. At the appointed time we reached her via phone. She was quite exhausted, she noted, from attending the office celebration that had prevented her from meeting with us earlier.

She informed us that one of our numerical measures did not meet their required threshold. We checked the measure, and the number we had supplied did, in fact, meet the threshold. She continued to insist that it did not. The issue, it turned out, was that our numerical result was in the form of a percentage, but our auditor had expected it to be in the form of a fraction (i.e., 40 percent vs. 4/10). Only with great effort were we able to explain the mathematical concept that the percentage and the corresponding fraction represented the same value, and that the value met their threshold. The auditor finally accepted our explanation, though I don't think we had her fully convinced. Still, we were required to amend our application. It was subsequently approved, and we were allowed into the pilot program. But the experience tarnished our view of the NCQA. We were answering to people who couldn't comprehend fractions!

What's Wrong with the PCMH Picture?

A full critique of the NCQA PCMH guideline could get mightily boring and overly wonky, so I will focus on just a few key areas. In addition, there are other PCMH models, so the strengths and weaknesses in this one may not be shared by all.

The NCQA's PCMH program is, more than anything else, just too much. The 2014 NCQA PCMH Standards and Guidelines weigh in at 93 pages, with an added 126 pages of appendices. All in all, the guidelines encompass 178 standards. That is too many. Where streamlined elegance is needed, overreaching is the rule. Where relief from the already crushing burden of bureaucracy is needed, more is being heaped on. And at a time that medical practices already struggle with expenses, this model promotes spending more money on administrative tasks and staffing. It is difficult to see how this will "revitalize the joy of practice."

It is important to ask why, in an era when administrative simplification is a recognized necessity that is even written into federal rulemaking guidelines (the Health Insurance Portability and Accountability Act, otherwise known by its abbreviation, HIPAA, includes an entire "Administrative Simplification" provision), we are still headed in the opposite direction. There is the desire when designing a program such as the PCMH to be thorough, transparent, and inclusive. In an effort to achieve this, it is standard practice to bring as many stakeholders as possible into the guideline-writing process. But then each stakeholder feels a need to add their two cents, and organizers likely shy away from removing anyone's input. So, the desire to be more open and democratic may encourage administrative bloat. And bloated it is—the NCQA PCMH model includes and codifies essentially every popular practice management fad of the twenty-first century, without regard for proven benefit.

Added to that is the notion that everything today must be measured. The mantra has become "How are you going to measure that?" It is the administrators' pledge of allegiance, and it is heresy to question the practice. And so, along with every standard, there must also be a way to document and measure compliance. Under such circumstances, it becomes especially challenging not to go overboard.

Here is the problem. Thorough documentation and meaningful data are essential aspects of a performance-improvement program, but dogmatic overreliance on them destroys such programs. A more balanced approach is needed to prevent compliance and data collection—rather than improved care—from becoming the focus. But the NCQA has clearly fallen into this common trap. There are actual times when one is forced to document time spent documenting. Compliance with the NCQA PCMH standards is so challenging that many practices hire extra staff to do it. The PCMH model acknowledges this, as many PCMH programs—our pilot program included— urge hiring "care managers," a vaguely defined new position deemed necessary to help administer the PCMH's many requirements.

A September 2015 article in *HealthIT Analytics* titled "Patient-Centered Medical Home Upkeep Costs $8,000 per Month" states that "maintaining PCMH certification can be an onerous and lengthy process, sapping even more time and energy away from over-burdened staff members." The article reports on a study of primary care practices in Utah and Colorado participating in the 2011 NCQA PCMH model. The study found that providers in Utah spent an average of $7,691 per month on PCMH personnel requirements, while Colorado providers spent $9,658 per month. Dr. Edward Bujold, a North Carolina family physician and participant in PCMH-related research activities, argues in this article that the PCMH, in conjunction with participation in programs such as Meaningful Use, has led him and his staff to spend "hundreds of hours studying for and taking exams, certifying for numerous programs, and updating then relearning our EHR to meet meaningful use requirements. . . . This was time we could have spent in patient care." The article also reports that Dr. Bujold "is considering walking away from the PCMH model due to its unreasonable administrative demands."

Such a critique raises a sensible question, though: How does a program like the PCMH assure compliance or judge performance with fewer requirements or less data? The answer, again, is that less may be more. To be of real value, a program like the PCMH must choose much more wisely what measures to include. It is much better for practices to achieve excellence and to thoroughly embody real change across a small number of key measures than to half-heartedly and temporarily make changes for this bloated, likely unsustainable model. And dare I say it—not everything needs to be measured.

Duplication and Dubious Requirements

It would be a simple matter to shorten the NCQA's guidelines because many of them duplicate the content of other programs, especially the previously critiqued, and super bad, EHR Meaningful Use program. By my analysis, about 30 percent of the PCMH written standards are a word-for-word duplication of the Stage 1 and 2 Meaningful Use requirements, many of which have been removed because they have been deemed inappropriate and excessive.

But also, many of the NCQA's requirements are just of dubious or unproven value, or prescribe one approach that may not represent the best or only way to get things done. For instance, the section on "team-based care" dictates that "the practice provides continuity of care for patients/families" by:

- Monitoring the percentage of patient visits with selected clinician or team
- Having a process to orient new patients to the practice
- Collaborating with the patient/family to develop/implement a written care plan for transitioning from pediatric care to adult care

149

While the concept of continuity of care (where patients get to see the same clinician over time) is of great value, monitoring data on such things is a questionable use of a practice's time. Requiring an orientation process for new patients? Give me a break. Requiring a written plan for the transition from pediatrics to adult care? In this written transition plan, it is suggested that one includes information covering "obstacles to transitioning to an adult care clinician," "information provided to the patient about the transition of care," and the "patient response to the transition." I think the program would live on without these requirements.

In the NCQA's "Performance Measurement and Quality Improvement" section is a measure that prescribes that "at least annually, the practice obtains feedback from patients/families on their experiences with the practice and their care." They must conduct a survey on at least three of the following categories:

- Access
- Communication
- Coordination
- Whole person care/self-management support

Oh, brother! These are the kinds of surveys that get administrators excited but take doctors and their practices further and further away from taking care of their patients.

Team-Based Care and Care Coordination: What Hath God Overwrought?

The PCMH model gets into the most trouble when, in addition to describing the type of care that patients should receive, it dictates exactly how that care must be delivered, in the form of "team-based care" and "care management." It is helicopter parenting where gentle guidance is far more appropriate.

There is definitely value in having well-trained staff with clearly defined roles and responsibilities. In addition, there is no rule that states that only doctors and nurses can be part of the care process. Every staff member can play an important part. But the NCQA mandates an approach to "team-based care" that is pure overkill. The guidelines specify that "the practice uses a team to provide a range of patient care services" by:

- Defining roles for clinical and nonclinical team members
- Identifying the team structure and the staff who lead and sustain team-based care
- Holding scheduled patient care team meetings or a structured communication process focused on individual patient care
- Training and assigning members of the care team to coordinate care for individual patients
- Training and assigning members of the care team to support patients/families/caregivers in self-management, self-efficacy, and behavior change

Administering such teams becomes another burden. I have been involved in a number of practice redesign programs that dictated team projects and watched as many practices failed because they did not have the training, expertise, the personnel, but especially the extra time necessary to make their team successful or to make such an approach sustainable. There are too many other ways, far simpler ways, to organize staffing and clinical care to dictate this particular approach. In our practice, we have a written training manual that thoroughly defines the practice's organization and every staff member's clinical and administrative responsibilities. All new staff receives thorough training. As a result, we function as an organized unit despite not having formalized teams or special team meetings (we talk about patients throughout the day), or providing anyone with data about such activities (required by the NCQA), which adds administrative burden, but little in the way of improving care.

A formal process of "care management" for complicated patients, those who tend to utilize the most health-care resources, is another popular, but overwrought and all too nebulous, concept mandated by the NCQA guidelines. Every medical practice has its well-known patient "high utilizers," frequent flyers in ERs and hospitals who cost the health system an inordinate amount of money. It is known that the costliest 1 percent of patients in the US account for 21 percent of all health-care expenditures, and that the top 5 percent generate 50 percent of the cost. The NCQA presumes that having every practice develop a new process, beyond the usual medical appointment, to identify such patients and to attempt to address each one's special needs and challenges will reduce their numbers and associated health-care expenditures. Practices are even urged to create a new staff position, the "care manager(s)," to guide and document this new process.

The NCQA PCMH guidelines specify that practices must "Identify Patients for Care Management," where "the practice establishes a systematic process and criteria for identifying patients who may benefit from care management. The process includes consideration of the following: (1) Behavioral health conditions, (2) High cost/high utilization, (3) Poorly controlled or complex conditions, and (4) Social determinants of health." Practices are instructed "to develop and update an individual care plan . . . for at least 75 percent of the patients identified."

My nurses, colleagues, and I keep scratching our heads on this one because we thought there was already a process in place to address patients' needs (even special needs) and to document their care—their appointments! We've always managed our patients' care and tried to address both their medical and nonmedical needs!

That's what I thought we were supposed to do during a medical appointment. I didn't make this up—that's exactly what I was trained to do in medical school and residency, and so we've always done it.

Let's assume, for the sake of argument, that my training and my practice represent some type of aberration, and that many physician practices don't provide such "care management." If that is the case, then we should be asking some basic questions. Number one is why? But we know the answer already. Doctors and their practices are too damned distracted by our dysfunctional medical system and burgeoning administrative and regulatory demands to do anything but the bare minimum. But that raises another question. Is the answer to fix the system and to retool the basic appointment, or to add yet another layer of administration and staffing, "care management" and "care managers," to try and bypass the whole mess?

Further, are we sure that formal "care management" and this new staff position, the "care manager," will necessarily lead to better outcomes? I am not convinced that such concepts are understood or studied to the point that they should be formally required of every practice, or that they would necessarily perform better than a high-functioning medical practice that provides comprehensive appointments. Once again, the helicopter-parent PCME model just goes way too far in mandating one approach.

High-needs patients can have extraordinarily complicated and challenging issues, in addition to their strictly medical ones (which are challenging in their own right), that run the gamut from poverty, to lack of education, to mental health and substance abuse issues, to lack of transportation, to joblessness and homelessness, to poor access to health-care resources, to loneliness, to the broad challenges of aging, and even just poor motivation. The list is endless and reflects growing inequality as well as the systemic weaknesses of the American social safety net and our lousy, fragmented health-care system—some of our greatest failures as a nation. In essence, we are asking doctors and their practices, through "care management," to stick their fingers in this crumbling dike, and we are assuming this will make a significant difference.

But there is little evidence that shows which "care management" interventions make a difference or how to proceed. Once a high-needs patient is identified, what is a practice to do, realistically, to reliably deliver better outcomes? And how much time, effort, and resources are reasonable or appropriate?

Using this "care management" philosophy, years back, my practice decided to take on our most challenging patients. It certainly seemed like the sensible thing to do. We would see these patients as frequently as necessary (once or twice weekly if need be) and work on fine-tuning both their medical and nonmedical issues. We educated. We identified community resources that might be of help and arranged for patients to receive such services (if they existed or seemed to be of value). We did, and still do, house calls for patients who could not come to us. We did whatever we could, and with great gusto I might add. There were some successes. But we also found that for some of these patients there was nothing we could do, and no extent we could go that made a substantial and reliable difference. Even with extreme effort, the results were unpredictable and often disappointing. We got the feeling that we would need to move in with some of these patients and take care of them full time if we expected to make any difference, but even that might not be enough. Our experience, and the lack of any real data to back these concepts or to guide such efforts, convinced me that requiring all practices to provide such formal "care management" and, especially, hiring care managers to do it should be questioned.

There may be effective ways to provide "care management" for high utilizers of care, but they likely involve profoundly different approaches and care models. There are, in fact, groups around the country that are beginning to develop such concepts and that are showing some signs of success, but their models involve a completely different level of care and involvement than might be reasonably expected—or even desirable—from a traditional medical practice.

One well-known and highly regarded group doing such work is the Camden Coalition founded by family physician Jeffrey Brenner, MD, to take care of Camden, New Jersey's, neediest patients. Since 2002, he has been developing a very sophisticated, data-driven, and innovative system of care to identify the highest-need patients and get them appropriate, timely, and coordinated care. Brenner stated in a 2014 interview, "The whole field of population health as an intellectual discipline is about thirty years behind where it needs to be. . . . We can separate Siamese twins, transplant hearts and lungs, cure some kinds of cancer, but we have no idea how to deliver better care at lower cost. . . . We don't have the basic research we need, and funding from the National Institutes of Health and AHRQ is lacking. We have a lot of incorrect models of care that don't work." What does appear to work involves things like going into patients' homes and diving deeply into their psychosocial needs. But as Brenner states, we need to "invest in building resources in communities that can deliver care to high-utilizing patients and others who need the most care.'

Until we understand such concepts better, have developed such resources, and can instruct physicians and their practices how best to proceed (and are willing to pay for such things), it is just premature and inappropriate to require that every practice add another layer of administration and staffing to become a veritable social services agency on top of everything else.

Until that time, the aim of programs like the PCMH should be to provide consistently excellent medical care to every manageable patient with chronic disease and to help practices foster an environment that promotes such things with specific tools and tips rather these heavy-handed requirements. The payoff would be large and more predictable.

In my practice, we pay exquisite attention to control of the most common chronic medical conditions, and we have seen the typical sequelae associated with these diseases—heart attacks, strokes, kidney failure, etc., almost disappear. We try extremely hard to stay on top of our "high utilizers," and go to some great lengths to do so, but also realize that there are limits to what we can accomplish with these cases in the current environment. We do our best.

And this brings me to my final criticism of the PCMH model. An excellent PCMH can still provide essentially lousy medical care. The PCMH model brings lots of extra bells and whistles to a practice, and even extra staff, but largely steers clear of the most important moment in patient care—the appointment. A well-run appointment between a clinician and a patient can and should result in most of what the PCMH model is trying to achieve. As I stated in this chapter's introduction, doctors are trained to provide the type of care prescribed by the PCMH model. We should attempt to refocus this key moment before we resort to more programs, more administration, and hiring more staff. The PCMH model, in effect, presumes that traditional appointments are a lost cause. It avoids the black box that is the exam room, where the nurse, the patient, and the clinician come together, and where almost all necessary care can and should take place.

Does the PCMH Model Work?

So what does the data show about the PCMH? Does the PCMH model improve performance and lower the costs of care? Not convincingly.

A systematic review of the effects of the PCMH model published in the February 2013 *Annals of Internal Medicine* concluded that "current evidence is insufficient to determine effects on clinical and most economic outcomes." The study found no cost savings and minimal impacts on clinical outcomes, though it was stated that "PCMH interventions had a small positive effect on patient experiences and small to moderate positive effects on the delivery of preventive care services. Staff experiences were also improved by a small to moderate degree."

A February 2014 Rand Corporation study reported in the *Journal of the American Medical Association* concluded that the PCMH model led to little improvement in quality and no reduction in use of services or total costs. The authors stated, "A multi-payer medical home pilot, in which participating practices adopted new structural capabilities and received NCQA certification, was associated with limited improvements in quality and was not associated with reductions in utilization of hospital, emergency department, or ambulatory care services or total costs over 3 years." They went on to conclude, "Despite widespread enthusiasm for the medical home concept, few peer-reviewed publications have found that transforming primary care practices into medical homes produces measurable improvements in the quality and efficiency of care."

One can find studies that show some limited benefits of the PCMH model, but the above results and the negative weight of most results make one wonder why CMS is making this unproven model one of the centerpieces of its new value-based payment system. Just as important, why do we let them get away with such things?

The Fix

So, doctors are taught to provide comprehensive care, but the realities of practicing in the American health-care system where they struggle just to get paid; where they battle against insurance companies hell-bent on denying patients' care; where they deal with unusable computer systems; and where they wrestle with insane, ever-changing government rules and regulations make doctors feel their only option is to churn out as many patients as possible. Everything else falls by the wayside.

And as this analysis shows, the bloated PCMH program further adds to the burden. It is just one more mess to deal with, and it hasn't been shown to be effective. And it doesn't change the fact that the rest of the health-care system is still broken. The PCMH program is like a Band-Aid placed over a huge gaping wound. It won't do much good unless we perform radical surgery to fix the underlying problems.

So, the first part of a solution would be to fix the health-care system rather than adding another layer of hassle and administration to the existing dysfunction. That's right, maybe if physicians practiced in a more cooperative, less distracting environment, they would be more apt to practice as they were trained. Maybe if they had more time during patient appointments, rather than less, things would be different.

More time, in fact, more than anything else might just be the key. The biggest impediment to making change in a medical practice is the constant pressure to see patients, to bring in revenue, and to keep up with burgeoning administrative demands.

How about, instead of adding to the burden, we pay physicians a lump sum so that they could take a half day per week away from direct patient care in order to focus on practice improvement? And how about, rather than requiring a host of unproven approaches, we provide doctors with a broad array of techniques that they could try, as they saw fit, to improve their practices?

Continuing the theme of increasing physicians' time with patients, part two of the fix would be to scuttle the harmful volume-based business model that most practices utilize and that encourages the shortest possible appointment times.

Believe it or not, there are ways to approach practice management other than throwing doctors onto the hamster wheel and turning up the speed every so often. One such practice model, known as the Ideal Medical Practice, focuses instead on lowering overhead expenses rather than maximizing patient volume. The hallmark of this approach is that lower overhead expenses make it so that physicians can see fewer patients without losing any money (they might even make more). Sounds too good to be true, doesn't it? But my own practice uses a version of this approach very successfully.

I use a brief math exercise to illustrate how the model works: Assume for this exercise that a physician is paid $70 per patient appointment. Based on that, we can calculate that for each patient we see in a day we will generate approximately $17,000 a year (you can take my word for it). A traditional practice employs 3.5 to 7 staff per clinician, and salaries are the number one overhead expense in most medical practices. Let's assume an average employee costs a practice $40,000 per year, and that office expenses are $3,000 per month ($36,000 per year).

- Scenario #1: Traditional high-overhead practice; physician sees 16 patients per day and has 4 employees:
  - Annual Revenue: $272,000
  - Annual employee costs: $160,000
  - Annual office expenses: $36,000
  - Doctor take-home pay (revenue – expenses) = $76,000
- Scenario #2: Low-overhead practice; physician sees 16 patients per day and has 1 employee:
  - Annual Revenue: $272,000
  - Annual employee costs: $40,000
  - Annual office expenses: $36,000
  - Doctor take-home pay (revenue – expenses) = $196,000

Another way to look at it is that in a traditional practice, where there are four employees to one physician, it would take 23 patients per day (7 more patients per day) for the physician to earn the same amount as in the low-overhead approach. More patients need to be seen to keep up with higher overhead costs.

What is also apparent from the exercise is that in a low-overhead practice model, patient appointments can be longer. If a physician sees patients 7.5 hours per day, 16 patients spread over that time results in an average appointment time of over 28 minutes. In the higher-overhead scenario, where the physician sees 23 patients in a day, the average appointment is only 19 minutes. So the math demonstrates that in a low-overhead practice model, physicians can see fewer patients but earn the same amount, and patients can have longer appointments.

The implications of such a model are profound. Most importantly, patients and physicians are much happier because each gets more time. In that extra time, a lot of great work—like comprehensive, holistic care—can take place! I can vouch for this model. It has worked very well for my practice.

How have we been able to lower our overhead, or in other words, gotten by with substantially fewer staff? We have reimagined the traditional staffing patterns most often used in medical practices, and we have used our technology creatively. It is traditional, in a primary care medical office, to have separate staff sit at the front desk, answering phones and checking in patients, to have nurses whose sole function is to bring patients to the exam room and register their vitals, and to have referral staff to arrange patient appointments with specialists, to name just a few of the usual support staff that help to run things. In our practice, we have one staff member, whom we call the super nurse, who does all those jobs at once. This staffing arrangement has worked very well for us even though we have far fewer employees.

The same techniques would work well in a larger organization, but they have one other huge source of overhead costs that might be reduced—administration. I did an analysis of an actual medium-sized health system that lists the names and salaries of its twenty top administrators. The average pay for these executives (positions like the Vice President for Medical Services, the Chief Information Officer, and the Vice President for Organizational Development) was roughly $500,000 per year (the CEO received much more), so the total amount spent on their salaries comes to about $10 million annually. By my analysis, it takes approximately 140,000 patient appointments (at $70 per appointment) to generate the revenue to cover these salaries every year. Another way to view this is that it takes almost twenty-eight physicians just to pay these executives (who generate little or no income, are paid far more than most physicians, and go to lots of meetings). Get my point?

So, in a better practice environment and using a more enlightened practice management model, physicians might just provide more comprehensive care without the need for an overly prescriptive program like the PCMH.

And in such an environment, a simplified PCMH-style guideline, one that uses a less prescriptive and less data-obsessed approach, might be of great value in shaping physician practices and the care they deliver.

CHAPTER 8

Getting Paid—Part 3: Holy MACRA

J ust to give you an idea of where things are headed here, alternate titles for this chapter include: "Getting Paid—Part 3: Armageddon"; "The Death of Reason"; and "You Think Climate Change Is Bad? Wait Till You See This!"

So, "Getting Paid—Part 1" focused primarily on how a doctor determines how much they can charge for an appointment. "Getting Paid—Part 2" was about how the payments flow (haphazardly) through the system. And in "Getting Paid—Part 3," we discuss how the government determines the amount it pays for physician services. I will give the government one thing when it comes to paying for health care—it is consistent—consistently, unbelievably bad!

Our story begins with an abbreviation that is akin to a bad word for doctors—"SGR." You want to start a fight with a doctor? Begin any sentence with "Your mother" and end it with "SGR." I don't care what's in the middle of that sentence, that doctor will come at you.

SGR stands for "sustainable growth rate," which refers to the method used by the Centers for Medicare and Medicaid Services since 1997 to determine the amounts Medicare pays to physicians for their services. The idea underlying the SGR was to keep annual Medicare spending increases below the annual growth in the gross domestic product. The SGR calculation was complicated, based on things like changes in the GDP, the previous year's payments to physicians, and the number of Medicare beneficiaries. The resultant SGR was then converted to the physician fee schedule using a calculation based on two factors: "1 plus the Medicare Economic Index (MEI)" and "1 plus the Update Adjustment Factor (UAF)." I don't know what either of those really means, but I suspect they are formulas with lots of variables, like x's and y's, where x stands for something like "stiff the doctors" and y stands for something like "stiff the doctors again." And in this respect—that is, stiffing the doctors—the SGR was quite effective.

I say that because, no matter what the GDP did from year to year (it typically has gone up a little each year), the SGR calculation tended to result in a huge reduction in physician fees. Between 2008 and 2009, during that wonderful time known as the Great Recession, the GDP went down about 2 percent. But, using the SGR conversion, physician fees were to be slashed a whopping 21.3 percent! The next year, the GDP rebounded, going up about 4 percent. Despite that, the calculation resulted in a fee reduction of an astounding 25 percent! Now, I am no mathematician, but it doesn't take one to know that these SGR conversions do not in any way reflect changes in the GDP.

Understandably, physicians would become somewhat upset each year when it was announced that Medicare payments, already so low compared to what most commercial insurers paid (Medicare pays approximately 80 percent of commercial insurances on average) that some physicians refused to see Medicare patients, were being cut further, and by such staggering amounts. No worries, though. Each time, Congress would intervene, and at the eleventh hour throw out the calculation and announce a corrected fee schedule.

It was a little disconcerting, though, thinking that your pay depended on an act of Congress. You know, Congress, that fun bunch best known for infighting, gridlock, and closing the government from time to time. It became an irritating and all-too-frequent ritual. The process even had its own name before long, the "doc fix." Prior to 2010, Congress made each "doc fix" prior to the deadline. But as political polarization grew, Congress became more and more sedentary. It began to miss the deadlines. On March 1, 2010, the physician fee schedule was slated to go down by 21.3 percent. On March 3, 2010, Congress enacted a delay in the pay reduction that lasted until April 1. That date came and went without a fix, which finally came on April 15, when they again made a temporary fix that would last only until June 1. But it wasn't until June 25 that another temporary fix was enacted, this one lasting until late November 2010. But at least the fix was retroactive to June 1. It suffices to say that this process was incredibly disruptive, one more huge distraction to physicians, who no longer knew if, when, or how much they were going to be paid. Nor did it inspire confidence in either our government or CMS.

Some people rationalize government inaction with phrases such as "democracy moves slowly," as if that is some sort of virtue. Well, if slow government is a virtue, then Congress was being especially virtuous because this painful process continued until April 2015, when they finally rose to the call, and with great fanfare did away with the evil SGR. They replaced this evil abbreviation with what would slowly become the next, even more evil, abbreviation, MACRA, the Medicare Access and CHIP Reauthorization Act of 2015.

Doctors were so desperate for change by this point, that they were willing to take just about anything, even a kick in the testicles, as long as it ended the SGR. And that was good, because that's what they got, only they didn't know it yet. The details of the new system emerged slowly. Beginning in 2019, doctors would begin to be paid not just for volume, but also for what is being referred to as value. That couldn't be so bad, right?

Doctors breathed a collective sigh of relief. First of all, 2019 was a way off. Except (surprise!) the program didn't really start in 2019. In typical government doublespeak, 2019 actually meant 2017, because the calculations that would determine payments in 2019 would be based on data collected for the year 2017. Most physicians didn't become cognizant of such things until sometime in 2016. Only at that point did the details of this new calculation begin to come into focus. And as those details became clear, many doctors began to be nostalgic for the once-hated SGR.

In a nutshell, CMS is taking every concept that has not worked over the past ten years—every fad, every unproven technique, and even some of its biggest failures—and rolling them all into one big sucker punch to medicine. Quality metrics? Yes, they're in there. Meaningful Use canceled? Maybe CMS said it was, but it's in MACRA. Penalties? Sure.

As part of MACRA, CMS has developed the Quality Payment Program, or QPP, which specifies two possible paths for physicians to be paid (or penalized) in the new system:

1. Merit-Based Incentive Payment System (MIPS)
2. Alternative Payment Models (APMs)

It's a lot more abbreviations to hate. MIPS is a new program where physicians will be rated over four areas: quality, resource use, clinical practice improvement activities, and meaningful use of certified EHR technology. Performance in the four weighted categories will result in the MIPS Composite Performance Score. Based on this score, physicians and practitioners will receive positive, negative, or neutral adjustments in their Medicare Part B base payment rate, eventually as much as 9 percent up or down.

One especially fun fact, as I mentioned earlier, is that each physician's performance will be compared to a national median, and if an individual's score is beneath the median, their pay will be reduced; if it is above the median, they will receive a bonus. In other words, no matter what, 50 percent of physicians in the MIPS program receive a penalty and 50 percent get a bonus. In other words, it is conceivable that a physician could perform well, even exceeding every standard, but still receive a penalty. That's what the government calls a budget-neutral program—any increase in costs is offset by an equal reduction. If I performed well, but still received a penalty, I would call that being screwed.

A brief critique of the MIPS four-pronged performance score is in order. In the quality performance category (50 percent of the total score), physicians will be required to report on six quality metrics. We discussed the drawbacks of this approach in Chapter 6, where we learned that use of quality metrics is an ineffective way to improve performance and results in disincentives to providing the best care.

For the resource use performance category (10 percent of the total score), CMS will calculate a physician's Medicare spending per beneficiary and the amounts spent on forty-one types of patient-care episodes for that physician, and compare those costs to those generated by other physicians. Obviously, this is a not-so-subtle incentive for physicians to withhold medical care from patients and to want to avoid the sickest patients who tend to generate the most costs. Imagine what might go through a physician's head, knowing they might receive a cut in pay if their patients cost the system too much, as they discuss treatment options with sick patients and their families. Did anyone say "death panels"?

For the clinical practice improvement activities (CPIA) category (15 percent of the total score), physicians can, as individuals or in groups, choose from ninety different practice improvement activities in six different categories, each worth up to 20 points. Full credit is achieved by scoring 60 points. One of the biggest struggles over the last few years has been trying to keep up with all of the different quality- and data-reporting programs. When CMS rolled out MACRA, it promised that it was easing the burden by combining everything into one program and reducing the number and types of requirements. But this is a completely new activity. Not much is known about the individual activities at this time.

And finally, we have the meaningful use of certified EHR technology category (25 percent of the total score). The Meaningful Use program, previously discussed, is in tatters. It is not yet clear how the new program will be structured.

Two things seem apparent. In an effort to get paid, doctors will be forced to chase a great deal of data and to participate in more projects, not fewer. This has the potential to be one more great big distraction, quite possibly the biggest so far, that takes clinicians even further from their focus on patient care. But also, by making penalties a standard aspect of the payment system, CMS will be penalizing the physicians who take care of the sickest patients. By establishing a penalty system based on the results of both quality metrics and "resource use," CMS will be encouraging bad care (doctors will feel the urge to meet numeric standards that are not appropriate for many patients), avoidance of the sickest patients (who have an adverse effect on quality metrics and who cost the most), and withholding of necessary care (physicians receive penalties if their care costs too much).

This was definitely on my mind during a recent appointment with a longtime patient, who, like many of my patients, has diabetes and is overweight. In preparation for the appointment, I was going through the patient's labs and noted that their HgbA1c, the most common measure used to assess diabetes control, had gone way up. When I saw the patient, I inquired what had happened. They chuckled and said, "I guess that bag of candy every day is a problem." It most assuredly is. But it's the kind of thing I hear throughout the day. In the past, I viewed moments like these as a part of my job that I relished. Patients like this need me, and I consider myself particularly good at getting such patients back on track, usually through some combination of lifestyle modification and medication changes. And my relationship with such patients is the key to my ability to spur successful behavior changes in such instances. But if I am going to receive a financial penalty for such patients, for things that may be beyond my control, it undermines that relationship. In fact, the more difficult the patient, and the less likely they are to hit their numbers, the less I might want them in my practice—the exact opposite of what we want. The system penalizes me for taking care of the patients who need help the most.

The second possible path under the MACRA program is for a physician to work within an Advanced Alternative Payment Model, or Advanced APM. The definition of what constitutes an Advanced APM is still somewhat hazy, so much so that CMS is establishing a Physician-Focused Payment Technical Advisory Committee to review and assess additional physician-focused payment models. Certain types of PCMH models will qualify as an Advanced APM. We discussed PCMHs in the last chapter. They entail a lot of work for physician practices and have not been shown consistently to effectively increase quality or lower the costs of care. So, of course, they are included.

A second type of care model that will satisfy this second MACRA track is a Next Generation Accountable Care Organization (ACO). An ACO is a health-care organization that receives payments that are tied to performance on quality metrics and its ability to control costs. At its most basic, an ACO combines capitated payments (capitated payments provide physicians a set amount for each patient for a specified period of time, usually a month, like the payment system that was used with the Health Maintenance Organizations of the

1990s) with the pay-for-performance concept, neither of which, as we've discussed in previous chapters, has been found to be effective.

Have ACOs been successful? It is a controversial topic. In an October 2015 article in *U.S. News and World Report* titled "Do Accountable Care Organizations Work?" Alice Rivlin, director of the Health Policy Center and Leonard D. Schaeffer Chair in Health Policy at Brookings Institution, commented, "So far the results have been very disappointing." Rivlin further explained that "while the drive to build ACOs to better coordinate care has arguably led some organizations to meet quality metrics, so much debate remains about the extent to which that translates to meaningful improvements in care for patients." And, she added, "ACOs haven't dented cost." To make a long story short, most of the articles I read on the topic of whether or not ACOs are successful concluded things like "experts disagree" or "the question has not yet been fully answered." It is odd, then, that CMS would make ACOs one of the centerpieces of its cost-cutting and performance-improvement efforts.

And there it is. CMS is replacing the failed, hated SGR with something that may be worse. Not one aspect of the various approaches being tossed into the new MACRA payment system has been proven to be effective. It is a giant gamble that promises to become a giant distraction for health care.

And here's the really funny part. None of the old system is actually changed. The crazy calculations necessary to compute how much a doctor can charge, described in "Getting Paid—Part 1," are still there. The insanity doctors go through to collect payments, detailed in "Getting Paid—Part 2," is unchanged. The data collection and new programs required under MACRA are in addition to everything else we have had to do historically to get paid!

So, physicians will still be paid for volume—with the largest part of their incomes still based on numbers of appointments and procedures—as it has been traditionally. In addition, now there will be an incentive to overprescribe and over-test in an effort to get patients to their numeric goals, no matter what is appropriate for the patient, and, at the same time, to withhold care so that resource use scores are low. MACRA creates a system that stumbles all over itself and that introduces, more than anything else, care confusion.

As of September 2016, the MIPS program is slated to begin in about three months, though it has yet to be fully defined in a CMS final ruling. So, ostensibly, physicians are going to be forced to participate, in very short order, in a program that includes drastic changes and will necessitate significant planning and restructuring with essentially no time to prepare. It's the government way!

The Fix

Each of the individual aspects of the MACRA program has been critiqued in previous chapters, so it is unnecessary to rehash old arguments. I would merely advise that CMS, whose recent track record has been so bad, not bite off so much more than it can chew. A much more limited and far more gradual approach would be appropriate. A better way forward, I think, is suggested in the next—and final—chapter.

CHAPTER 9

The Real Big Fix

Alas, it is time to wrap things up.

To begin with, there were certainly lots of other distractions I could have included in the book. It's worthwhile to give some of them at least a brief mention.

It is not that these topics have no value. First and foremost, I chose to write about what I know best. But I believe there is value in a more thorough analysis of the topics that I have not included. In fact, I would welcome it. Did anyone say sequel?

Second, I chose to focus on areas with which people are less familiar and that are largely absent from the public discourse on health-care reform, though absolutely crucial to its success. Without a better understanding of these issues and their implications, we will continue to blunder along. I also believe I have presented this information in a unique way, one that makes the problems clearer and solutions more obvious. I am confident that the book's themes hold true, and that the lessons we can draw provide a better way forward for health care. And the "fixes" at the end of each chapter provide commonsense, workable solutions. They are intended as the beginning of a conversation, though, not the end.

I would also note that the information I have presented tends to be outpatient-focused. There are lots of terrible goings on within hospitals and large health systems that I did not discuss. I work as an outpatient primary care physician, and the topics I included, and my biases, reflect my experiences more than anything else.

I have not touched upon the Health Insurance Portability and Accountability Act (HIPAA), the obese set of government rules that, as they are understood by most people, are intended to protect the privacy and security of patients' health information. Most people even think that the *P* in the HIPAA abbreviation stands for "privacy." But the ruling, updated in 2013, actually deals with a huge number of other issues including protection of health insurance coverage for employees when they change or lose jobs, and—somewhat comically—an entire section devoted to administrative simplification. To most health-care professionals, "HIPAA" is a dirty word that represents the opposite of administrative simplification. Ironically, because of HIPAA, I have had hospital staff question if it is appropriate to discuss my own patients' care with me! One patient recently told me that he was forbidden to view his own wrist x-ray due to HIPAA.

Another patient's cancer care was held up because her oncologist was unable to obtain the results of testing that had been done at another facility. So as a result of the HIPAA ruling, so much emphasis has been placed on privacy, and threats of legal action and penalties for violating one of the rule's complicated requirements are so great, that medical professionals are too frightened to share needed information with one another. So, in its effort to protect health information, HIPAA impedes its flow. The bottom line is that the HIPAA rules are so dense, and compliance so challenging, that they defeat their own purpose.

Nor did I discuss one of the most distracting of the distractions—Maintenance of Certification (MOC), the criminally stupid and expensive hoops that doctors are forced to jump through in order to maintain their licensure and professional certification. Traditionally, to be "certified," doctors have to obtain a certain number of continuing medical education credits every year and to periodically take and pass official board exams. In recent years, however, the certifying agencies (mine is the American Board of Family Medicine, the ABFM) have markedly expanded the requirements and increased the costs. They have devised all manner of new testing modules and time-consuming practice improvement projects. For instance, I had to compile and submit data about how many times my staff and I washed our hands while we saw patients. To receive credit for my efforts, I had to pay hundreds of dollars. Each new requirement comes with a mandatory fee. It is abusive, redundant (there are similar performance-improvement activities associated with participation in the PCMH program and the new MACRA payment program), and of questionable value. Fed up, physicians have begun to rebel. Some are even choosing to boycott the process altogether. In response, the certifying agencies have pledged to make improvements. In fact, recently I received a notification from the ABFM detailing the changes. In perfect bureaucratic form, none of the requirements were changed but each of them appears to have been given a new name! Cheeky bastards!

And, of course, I have not discussed the need to reform our medical malpractice system. Because of the ever-present threat of litigation, every physician today practices some version of "defensive medicine," otherwise known as "cover your ass" (CYA). We order extra tests and overtreat for fear that any mistake, delay, negative outcome, or other perceived slight will result in a multimillion-dollar lawsuit. It is an unbalanced and ineffective system that increases health-care costs in the name of huge settlements and legal fees, as opposed to improved patient care.

And then there's the oft-evil pharmaceutical industry. Outlandish prescription prices bring to light the moral hazards of a corporate culture that values shareholder profits over everything else. Mylan CEO Heather Bresch rationalized increasing the price of the EpiPen 400 percent, which is essentially the attempted murder of poor people with allergies, by saying, "I am running a business." Apparently this is code for "I have no soul." I run a business, too. There's a big difference between being successful and making money, and killing people to do it! Rulings by the US Supreme Court have created the notion that corporations are people. If that is so, then many pharmaceutical corporations are bad people. When Gilead Science prices the hepatitis C drug Harvoni at $84,000, and when Novo Nordisk makes Levemir insulin too expensive for diabetics to afford, then patients do not get readily available, necessary, and lifesaving treatments. They suffer and die as a result. It highlights the need for government regulation, *good* government regulation, to protect citizens from the harmful consequences of uncontrolled corporate greed. The American government could and should use its power to negotiate cheaper prescription prices. Oh, and enjoy hell, Heather.

This final section of *Distracted* is intended to bring things together. In the first part, we will review and flesh out the book's themes. We then go to a crucial topic—broken government and bad bureaucracy—the crux of what is wrong with American health care. In this brief section, we examine the problems and suggest a fix. We then take on traditional aspects of health-care reform, informed and reinterpreted by what we have learned. We will fix the main problems: access to care, cost of care, and quality of care.

And finally we must ask how we ensure that any of this comes to pass. How do we derail a government and a health-care administrative system that does not budge? With a government now defined by gridlock and an all-powerful corporate machine holding the reins of power, is there a way that we can make any of these changes a reality? It is one of the central questions of the twenty-first century, and one that pertains to all industries, not just health care. If we don't find an answer to this question, then all of this has just been an intellectual exercise. And American health care will continue to sicken.

What We Can Conclude

The devil is in the details, and those details can make or break any approach to health-care reform. Doctors and nurses are treated the way Lucy treats Charlie Brown in the famous football gag scene. Lucy bullies and cajoles Charlie Brown until he finally agrees to kick the ball again, but inevitably, she yanks the ball away at the last second. Charlie Brown whiffs and falls on his ass. It's a setup every time.

In modern health care, we badger medical professionals to improve performance but then force them to participate in a myriad of ineffective mandatory programs, withhold the tools they need to attain the goals we set out for them, often block them from providing the best health care, and then penalize them when they fail.

Doctors are bogged down by crazy calculations, confusing codes, and arbitrary rules, packaged within a cumbersome and error-prone medical billing maze. Transactions that would take place as an afterthought in a world that made sense get sent to a dystopian billing nightmare so bad it could form the basis of a Terry Gilliam movie (see *Brazil*). It is clear that a simplified, working payment system would save health-care dollars and relieve doctors of an incredible burden and a pointless source of distraction.

We have also discussed how doctors have been forced by government mandate to purchase expensive, unusable EHR computer systems that frequently do not work and only rarely deliver on the great promise represented by health information technology. Rather than saving time, increasing income, and improving performance, as it was presumed they would, EHRs have forced many doctors to work longer hours, have wreaked havoc on practices' bottom lines, and have created an entirely new set of problems and challenges often worse than the ones associated with the paper records they replaced. The Meaningful Use program, possibly the federal government's hardest kick to the groin of medicine so far, has been more of a technology setback than a move toward the future. And still, nothing is clearer than the need for all physicians and nurses to have an affordable, usable, fully interoperable EHR program. We should expect little until we have such a program in every office and every hospital in America.

Next, we explored many of the ways that our insurance-based health-care system just does not work. There are still almost 30 million people without any insurance at all. But some who have insurance might argue that they are worse off than those who don't. Health insurance in the current era often carries exorbitant premiums, and many new policies have high deductibles, narrow and incomplete coverage, and prohibitive prior authorization procedures that keep patients from obtaining care, and require an entirely new set of skills for physicians forced to work around these barriers to care.

These crucial details are the difference between a functional health-care system and the disastrous one we have now. In other words, a simplified and improved medical billing and payment system, having affordable twenty-first-century health information technology in the hands of all physicians, and removal of the systematic barriers to care inherent in our current health insurance system are the very building blocks of health-care system success.

Before we can successfully move to improved models of care, like the PCMH, to sophisticated data-driven performance improvement, or to more value-based payment models, we must first fix these issues. Until we do this, making significant improvements in the American health-care system will be almost impossible. We will continue to fail, like Charlie Brown in the football gag.

These same details will make or break any approach to health-care reform. A single-payer system, the darling of many health-care activists and a system used successfully by other countries around the world—even though it is widely purported to streamline health care and lower costs—could be just as bad as the system we have now if we do not properly define the details and address the issues mentioned in this section. For instance, even if we are just dealing with a single payer—Medicare in this instance—if that single payer tightens the specificity requirements for diagnostic codes (as it is currently planning to do) too much or alters how doctors are paid for chronic care in some confusing new fashion (it is currently working on this issue), it may be just as hard for doctors to get paid. In addition, even in a single-payer system, Medicare could, in an effort to control costs further, expand prior authorization requirements to include more testing and more prescriptions (which it is currently doing, as well), which could result in more barriers to care than we have now.

I could also see how a multi-payer system like the one we have now, properly regulated and constructed to expand access and affordable care to all, could function much better with the above issues properly settled.

So, this gives us our priorities for the first part of true and transformative health-care reform:

1. A profoundly simplified, workable system of medical billing
2. Affordable, usable, interoperable EHR systems in the hands of all practicing physicians

3. Removal of systematic barriers to care, such as high deductibles, narrow and incomplete coverage, and restrictive prior authorization processes

Health care is not broken—it is the *administration* of health care that is broken. One of the key points brought to light in *Distracted*, and a very important point of departure from the usual conversation regarding American health care, is that it is not really "health care" that is failing. It is the *administration* of health care that is failing more than anything else. Medical professionals could be doing so many miraculous things today if only they functioned within a system that enabled and encouraged such things.

This is not to imply that doctors and the medical profession itself are without blame and do not share in the responsibility for what is wrong with American health care. Doctors make mistakes. It happens too often, and it is something for which we must take responsibility and for which we should be held accountable. The high rate of medical errors and suboptimal care is a troubling problem that needs to be addressed and that I believe can be improved upon and even fixed quite easily in many instances. The problem is that this is nearly impossible when doctors and nurses must devote more and more time to attempting to comply with new and ever-changing government mandates and they are forced to work within the constraints of a health insurance system that systematically keeps patients from receiving care. The sad fact is that many aspects of patient care, and the time and effort we could devote to improving patient care, take a backseat to navigating in and around the increasingly complicated and ever-changing health-care bureaucracy.

In such a system, doctors and nurses are becoming increasingly distracted and demoralized. But the greatest shame of all is that many are so troubled by what is happening that they are considering their options to leave what was not just a career, but a true calling.

But once again, a real understanding of the issues is the necessary first step toward a solution. It is clear that to successfully reform American health care, we need to drastically change how we administer the system. We need a less intrusive and more effective bureaucratic methodology and a balance of who controls health care and medical decision-making that includes patients and doctors.

Both government and the private sector are the problem. The typical conversation regarding health-care reform in America most commonly pertains to who pays for health care and how that system should be organized, and the argument usually pits government versus the free market (meaning the private sector), or some amalgam of the two, which of course is how our current system is organized (though "organized" might be a bad term to use under the circumstances). The battle lines are usually drawn along fairly strict and painfully polarized political divisions.

Republican politicians, pundits, and other right-leaners hold government in particularly low esteem (they are self-hating politicians). Not surprisingly, they tend to view government's involvement in health care as the problem. It is their view that only competition in a "free market" is capable of fixing what is wrong. If they have a leader, it is probably Senator Paul Ryan (R-Wisconsin), and if he has a plan, it is primarily to abolish Obamacare. Beyond that, he recommends a vague mix of tax credits and subsidies to defray the costs of health insurance, and essentially pushes everyone away from the government side of medical care, Medicare and Medicaid, toward private insurance.

That's all pretty hard to swallow, though, and it just doesn't line up with any version of reality that I am familiar with. As we have seen, our insurance-based system has failed to provide affordable health care for a huge percentage of Americans, and having health insurance is no longer the equivalent of having health care. And by pulling out of the Obamacare insurance exchanges, the health insurance industry is making it obvious that they will not be able to provide the comprehensive solution that American health care needs.

On the other side of the political spectrum, somewhere left and center of the Republicans, Democrats typically say that government is the answer, or at least part of the answer. They are proud of Medicare for its efficiency and for the fact that it provides access to health care for almost all seniors. Many favor retaining our "unique" mishmash of government-private-payer health care. They go to great lengths to try and show that Obamacare is working, though flawed, and suggest that what we need to do is to gradually build upon its successes. They point out that millions more people have been able to obtain health insurance since the advent of Obamacare but ignore just about everything else. They also seem essentially oblivious to the fact that, as this book points out time and again, government regulation is sucking the life out of health care.

Even further to the left (but sometimes from the center and even right) there are calls for the complete elimination of commercial health insurance in favor of a single-payer system. It should be noted that the term "single payer" describes the funding mechanism, but does not necessarily define the form of the health-care delivery system. A single-payer system would clearly place the reins even more firmly in the hands of government bureaucrats who are currently running roughshod over our health-care system and rarely like to pay for things without asking for a great deal in return.

And this is about as far as the typical conversation usually goes. But it ignores the great big elephant in the room, which is the obvious fact that, if you are really paying attention, it is clear that both government and the private sector are at fault when it comes to what is wrong with American health care. In other words, neither the government nor private insurance is doing a good job.

But if both government and the insurance companies are to blame, can we confidently point to either one as the solution? When you look at it that way, it makes things a little more difficult, doesn't it? We usually think in terms of those two entities in an either/or sense. But if both are the problem, then where can we turn?

The answer is that an entirely different approach just might be needed. Based on what we've just learned, I think there is a logical path forward. The number one priority, as I already pointed out, is to put in place the building blocks of health-care system's success. We also clearly need bureaucratic reform if we hope to end the current vicious cycle we are in. At that point, we can then take on the more traditional aspects of health-care reform: access to care, cost of care, and quality of care. But as we do that, we must take into account that both government and the private sector may pose problems, and undo our efforts, if we are not exceedingly careful how we proceed.

Bureaucratic Reform

I will point out from the outset that I am not anti-government. But I am decidedly anti-bad government, and likewise, I am pro-good government, though that seems to be in short supply these days.

And I am no political scientist, so I won't pretend too much to be one. As I like to say, I am but a simple country doctor. But this country doctor knows that the bureaucracy is broken and that broken bureaucracy is destroying the practice of medicine, and therefore, bureaucratic reform is the crux of health-care reform. It is unlikely that we will get one without the other.

But once again, the national conversation misses the point. We spend our time arguing about the size of government and the merits of more regulation versus deregulation. Though the government's large size is an obvious symptom of its dysfunction, it does not automatically follow that less government would be more functional government. The right size of government is that which effectively and efficiently achieves the objectives we set for it.

So, first we must discuss the appropriate role of government. Then, we have to discuss a more effective method to get the job done. The right size follows, and the number and size of regulations would almost assuredly be reduced. So, what is government's role supposed to be? I think it should simply be—to help.

Government's role in health care should be to help patients get the best care possible and to help medical professionals provide that care. But in doing so it must tread more lightly. It must practice a great deal more restraint. It should use the smallest tools necessary to get the job done. Getting the balance right is not easy.

The government I have described in *Distracted* seeks not to help but to control. The difference is palpable. This is clearly demonstrated in the billing and coding regulations discussed in "Getting Paid—Part 1." The government that wrote those types of regulations was (and still is) forcing doctors to obey its dictates, a far cry from helping them deliver better care.

And it marked a turning point for the practice of medicine—the era of distraction—where the government began to use more and more detailed regulation to force doctors to do exactly what it wanted, down to the minute details of practicing medicine.

The government's tool of choice became prescriptive regulations—regulations that force us at every critical juncture to turn in the direction of their choosing. Prescriptive regulations force doctors to write a clinical note, to use a computer, to prescribe a medicine, or to order a test in a particular manner, though often not the best manner.

But there are relatively few instances in something as complex as the practice of medicine where it is possible or desirable to prescribe the behaviors appropriate to every circumstance. As we have seen, prescriptive regulation does not enable the flexibility or the discretion necessary to navigate the reality of such situations. Moreover, it is an approach that almost by definition results in too much regulation. It has left us overloaded with rules that we can barely digest or comprehend and with which we struggle to comply.

A good deal of thought has been directed toward redesigning government. The Better Regulation Task Force, an independent organization that advises the British government, in 2003 published guidelines entitled *Principles of Good Regulation*. Refreshingly, the document is only ten pages—they practiced what they preached!

The guidelines caution that "where regulation is poorly designed or overly complicated it can impose excessive costs and inhibit productivity. The job of government is to get the balance right." It states that "policy-makers have a wide range of options available for implementing policy objectives. The Task Force urges them to consider them all, rather than automatically assume prescription regulation is required." The Task Force lists a number of alternative options that include doing nothing (my favorite); advertising campaigns and education: using the market; financial incentives; and self-regulation and voluntary codes of practice.

When it comes to most of the regulations that have been discussed in *Distracted*, "doing nothing" would almost always have been the better choice. Government should stand as far back as possible from clinical care. It should not be government's role to tell me how to write a clinical note, how or when to communicate with my patients, or how often to provide educational materials to them. I am quite capable of those things. I am a highly trained professional, with many years of schooling and now also many years of experience to hone my medical decision-making skills. On top of that, over time I get to know most of my patients and become familiar with their special circumstances. While I am all-too fallible, and I do make mistakes, I do not believe there are many instances where inflexible rules or arbitrary regulations will do better than me when

185

push comes to shove in the exam room. In other words, unless it is absolutely necessary, stay the hell out of my clinical practice.

The Task Force report also includes a policy-maker's checklist, detailing what "regulators should bear in mind" when devising regulations, including the concepts of proportionality ("intervene when necessary. Remedies should be appropriate to the risk posed."); accountability ("regulators must be able to justify decisions, and be subject to public scrutiny"); consistency; transparency; and targeting ("regulation should be focused on the problem, and minimize side effects"). To their list, I might add brevity and simplicity. Streamlined, elegant regulation is more likely to be effective regulation. New regulations should also be judged on their potential to simplify and reduce administrative demands. And finally, being the year 2017, we should subject all new regulation to a technology review to determine what aspects of implementation, compliance, and oversight could be automated, potentially freeing us even further from administrative consequences.

Philip K. Howard, in his book *The Rule of Nobody*, suggests a different direction for American regulators—to regulate by general principles instead of detailed rules in most instances. He states that "regulation by principles creates a starkly different way of making public choices. Instead of a legal instruction manual, public choices on what is sensible must be made by a person on the spot." Principles provide guidance and a framework within which to work, but the details, the judgments, and the ultimate decisions are left to those who know the situation best—in health care, that is the doctors, nurses, and their patients.

While doctors bristle at the mention of a Meaningful Use program that dictates the content of almost every aspect of their computerized charting, I think most would be fine with principles that established the general expectations for such things.

So, a better and more effective approach to regulating health care would be to use a range of options—less invasive approaches, such as principles, education, financial incentives, and ad campaigns for most matters—and more invasive rules and regulations only when absolutely necessary.

Over the years, CMS has given physicians and other health-care professionals many burdensome tasks. Now I have one for CMS. For the American health-care system to improve, CMS itself must be thoroughly redesigned. Its mission must become "to help patients get the best care possible, and to help medical professionals provide that care," and all of its efforts must be organized around that concept. All existing projects should be suspended and a moratorium should be placed on every new one. Every existing regulation must be rethought, rewritten, streamlined, or just plain gotten rid of using criteria like those mentioned above. And the top priority must be to put in place the building blocks of a successful health-care system, as detailed earlier in this chapter.

I will finish this section by acknowledging the elephant in the room—money in politics. Bad regulatory methodologies are not the only reason that government does not work. This government has thrown out, trampled on, or just ignored every concept of conflict of interest, morality, and even decency in how it has allowed and encouraged the undue influence of money to highjack its purpose. It is clear that this is no longer a government by and for its people, but one that is by and for those with the most money. The money and its influence are dominant throughout our government. Until this situation changes, there is little hope that CMS or our health-care system will be reorganized around the interests of patients and health professionals.

Improving Access to Care

Of all the flaws apparent in the administration of American health care, lack of access to care is still the biggest and the most far-reaching.

187

Our current insurance-based health-care system is clearly not working—many Americans are denied access to readily available care, and because of that, people needlessly suffer and die. It is an ugly stain on the American flag.

What every American needs, and must demand, is full access to affordable, comprehensive medical care. At a minimum, the system must include everyone, place a reasonable cap on all medical expenses, and cover a nationally determined comprehensive basket of medical goods and necessary services. In a sense, I don't care how it happens, as long as it does happen. This must form the basis of health-care reform, no matter the model. If America wants to be a great nation, it must guarantee access to care for its people.

Lowering the Costs of Care

There are two areas of focus pertaining to health-care expenditures—administrative costs (or the nonmedical costs) and the medical costs.

It is estimated that almost one-third of every dollar spent on health care in the United States represents nonmedical administrative costs. And after reading the "Getting Paid" chapters, you have a good idea where much of that money is going—medical billing hell. An overly complicated multi-payer system is a wasteful, expensive system.

A single-payer system is the best way to reduce health-care administrative expenditures because it reduces the number of payers to one. I will play devil's advocate, however, and caution that the number of payers is only one of the factors that make medical billing so complicated, and so wasteful, in the current system. As we learned, another important factor is the insane rules dictating how much doctors are paid, the confusing sets of billing and diagnostic codes, and the multistep billing process currently in place. A single-payer system does not necessarily eliminate any of this. In fact, it places firm control of the billing and payment system in the hands of the government bureaucrats that devised the system in the first place

Therefore, once again, we must define the details properly to ensure that any approach to health-care reform is successful. So, if we want the full reduction in administrative costs possible under a single-payer system, we must greatly simplify all processes that relate to getting paid. As stated earlier in this section, this is one of the building blocks of health-care system success.

But I think it is also valid to ask whether we could take a similar approach with the current multi-payer system? I think it would be much more difficult, but I could envision a multi-payer system with one set of simplified administrative rules and payment/billing processes that might offer savings similar to that of a single-payer system.

As for the medical costs (the non-administrative costs) of health care, I think, once more, that we are mostly missing the boat. Current approaches to lowering medical costs focus on limiting care (but it is often necessary care), using such tools as prior authorizations and restrictive medication formularies, or reductions in pay for physicians whose patients cost the system too much. As I've shown repeatedly, the current approach causes far more harm than good.

There is a much better, more sensible way to reduce health-care expenditures in the United States. According to the Centers for Disease Control and Prevention (CDC), "eighty-six percent of all health care spending in 2010 was for people with one or more chronic medical conditions." Chronic diseases such as cardiovascular disease and diabetes are the number one determinant of health-care costs in the United States. But such conditions are largely preventable. The combination of healthy eating, regular exercise, weight control, and avoidance of tobacco and excessive alcohol reduces mortality from heart disease, the number one killer in the nation, by 80 to 90 percent.

So, the number one opportunity to reduce health-care costs in the US is prevention of chronic disease through healthy living. And research has shown a substantial return on investment for employee wellness programs. So, if we really want to reduce health-care expenditures, we must develop a comprehensive national health and wellness system, and improve the health of the nation. Schools and places of work, where most people spend the greatest part of their day, should be incentivized to encourage and even provide options for healthy eating, and to provide time, every day for every student and employee, to engage in structured physical activity. A full-throttled push to improve the health of the nation would do far more to lower the costs of health care than any of the approaches previously discussed. And such an approach has no conflicting incentives to deny needed medical care. It is good for everyone.

Improving the Quality of Medical Care

We touched on this topic in the chapter "Measuring the Quality of Medical Care Is Bad for You," but focused primarily on how clinical quality measures could be better utilized to create a comprehensive system of performance improvement. I will reiterate one point from that section. Doctors and nurses need, more than anything else, time—time away from patient care and fewer hassles during patient care (but more time for each patient) if we expect them to find and implement performance-improvement solutions and successfully execute them in practice.

In this section, we will discuss other approaches we might use to improve the quality of American medical care.

The first of such approaches are work instructions and check-lists. In every practice improvement project in which I have been involved, it was emphasized that every medical practice, and every health system, is unique. and therefore, each must determine its own path to delivery of improved medical care.

As a result, individual practices receive little guidance regarding best practices in managing their offices or the delivery of medical care. Each practice, and every health system, must invent and reinvent this wheel, largely on their own. Unfortunately, what I have seen is that many practices have little idea how to proceed on their own, nor adequate time to devote to such efforts.

But the idea that every practice is different is also mostly wrong. The majority of what transpires in most medical practices, emergency rooms, and hospitals is the same. It repeats over and over, so it is patterned and almost entirely predictable. What this means is that we can, and should, devise and document best practices and processes that can be used to guide and to train all medical personnel to handle almost every circumstance.

In fact, I developed such written "work instructions" for my community clinic, and using them, we were able to transform our practice environment from one of confusion to one of reliability and excellence. These "work instructions" simply defined (in writing) the general expectations of each staff member during any type of patient encounter and the other common aspects of patient care. Knowledge became much more standardized across the organization and performance improved dramatically. I have colleagues who have embraced a similar approach and achieved similar results.

This simple but incredibly effective approach is similar to the checklists that Dr. Atul Gawande describes in his well-known book *The Checklist Manifesto: How to Get Things Right*. Gawande argues, "We need a different strategy for overcoming failure . . . and there is such a strategy—though it will seem almost ridiculous in its simplicity. . . . It is a checklist." Gawande describes scenarios where checklists have been used to markedly reduce infection rates, improve pain control, and reduce ventilator-related deaths. I believe that we could see similar results in office practices by developing various types of work instructions and checklists.

In our practice, we realized that with our rural location we were more likely to see patients with acute emergencies. The emergency that frightened me the most was anaphylaxis, a severe allergic reaction which, if incorrectly treated, can easily result in death. Early in my career, I lay awake more than a few nights mentally reviewing what I would do if such an emergency presented in my office. But I also worried that in an emergency I might forget some crucial step. And there was no guaranteeing that my staff would know what to do, either. So I wrote a one-page instruction, "Office Emergency Protocols," that listed the twelve most common office emergencies and provided a brief instruction detailing the treatments for each. The list was posted on the wall of each of our clinical rooms. These instructions have saved many lives, and we have successfully treated every one of the many serious anaphylaxis cases we have seen since this checklist was posted.

Checklists and work instructions can be used in almost every aspect of clinical care. Especially with the advent of more sophisticated EHR software, we can generate, in most common clinical scenarios, simple reminders and prompts, very similar to checklists, to trigger and encourage appropriate care.

Another way we could improve performance is by rethinking some of our traditional care delivery models. Take health maintenance, such as cancer screenings and immunizations, for instance. In the traditional care model, mammograms, pap smears, colon cancer screening, and the huge number of required immunizations are all the responsibility of individual physicians and their practices. The work involved is substantial.

But in light of the new and improved capabilities made possible by information technology, we could be providing and monitoring these important aspects of patient care in completely different and better ways. For instance, cancer screenings could be managed by a central agency that would receive all test results, generate timed reminder emails and calls, and even schedule further testing. With all of the demands on a modern clinician's time, we would be delighted to have such an option available to us. As long as practices continue to receive results of all such testing (as they always have), they can also serve as a backup, so that when patients are seen in the office, they can be notified of any noted gaps in care.

Another possible way to improve the quality of medical care would be more standardized and affordable continuing medical education (CME). As mentioned previously in this section, physicians are required to obtain a specified number and type of CME credits every year, and also to complete a burgeoning number of other time-consuming and costly tasks in order to maintain their certifications and licensure. Unfortunately, in spite of those requirements, and sometimes because of them (they are often of low quality), it is possible to have lots of CME credit but little to show for it. It is a shame that there is no one reliable source to which a physician can turn to review bread-and-butter medical care, new care guidelines, and recent developments in the medical sciences. Something as basic as a high-quality, comprehensive, and affordable source of CME tied to a streamlined maintenance of certification process might translate into better medical care.

Conclusion

And that gets us to the last, but maybe the biggest, question. Health care in America is broken in large part because government in America is broken. But finding, agreeing on, and implementing a comprehensive fix for the American government has been elusive. The twenty-first century has seen eight years of a Republican president followed by eight years of a Democratic president, and things have only gotten worse.

The only thing that is clear is that change does not appear to be coming from the top. We, the American people, must put aside those things that have traditionally divided us and come together to demand better from our so-called leaders and the government institutions that are supposed to exist by and for us all.

The same is true for health-care professionals—the doctors, nurses, and other medical personnel being sickened by this toxic work environment. We must find our voice, and unify and organize in entirely new ways to demand and shape a better environment for our patients and for us.

For health-care professionals, maybe the answer lies in traditional labor organizing, something that historically has been uncommon for physicians. I was recently contacted by a doctor friend, Cathy Maslen. We trained in the same residency program and have remained in touch since. Dr. Maslen has worked most of her career at a Baltimore-based community health center that catered to the medical needs of the gay and transgender community, as well as the inner-city poor. Cathy and her colleagues deal with some of the most challenging issues in all of medicine, and they do it with an uncommon commitment.

Unfortunately, new management at the health center, coupled with the destructive forces of the greater health-care system, is making their jobs even more difficult. In response to rising financial pressures, management has cut staff through multiple rounds of layoffs. Physician salaries have been cut 20 percent, though they can gain back that amount by seeing higher numbers of patients and through compliance with burdensome government data collection efforts and "quality" initiatives. The result is that the clinical staff is being pushed to do much more with much less, and they feel that patients are being endangered as a result.

So, they did something that doctors don't normally do. They contacted a local labor union and attempted to organize themselves. Management was not happy. They brought in strike busters. They pressured staff to vote against the union. They fired five longtime staff members who were accused of helping to organize the movement. That was a mistake. That really pissed off their patient community. It also caught the attention of the Baltimore media, which began daily coverage of the unfolding drama.

Patients organized a Friday evening protest attended by about a hundred community and staff members. Patients spoke in incredibly touching terms about what the fired staff members had done for them and meant to them over the years. They demanded their return.

The vote was held and the union was voted in. My hope is that this was one of the opening salvos in a battle where health-care professionals, and their patients, fight to take health care back.

The status quo in health care is killing us, literally. We the people must put a stop to it. We can easily have a working health-care system—accessible to all; affordable for everyone; and able to provide safe, high-quality, coordinated care for all. But the government won't do it. Corporations—the insurance companies and the pharmaceutical companies—won't do it. They are the problem, and they have so far been unable, unwilling, or both, to fix things, to stop the killing. So it is up to us.

Afterword: After Obamacare?
Probably a Lot Like Obamacare

T he only constant in life is that politicians talk about the need
for change.

Most of the content of *Distracted* was written in the
spring and summer of 2016, prior to the presidential election. Then
came the shocking victory of Donald Trump. The new president
and the Republican congressional majority immediately announced
their plans to throw out the singular embodiment of all they felt
was wrong with the previous administration: the Affordable Care
Act/Obamacare (it seems necessary to mention both the official
name and the nickname of former-president Obama's signature
health-care legislation, as recent reports have revealed that much of
the American population does not know that they are one and the
same). Since then, the push to repeal Obamacare has taken on an air
of near-religious fervor among Republicans.

It seemed appropriate then to add this brief section to *Distracted*
in anticipation of a world after Obamacare.

First of all, *Distracted* is primarily a critique (a distinctive one)
of the negative impacts of Obamacare-era health-care administration and regulation, so as the nation continues to argue about the

proper path forward to fix American health care, that aspect of the book remains extremely relevant. And second, and maybe more importantly, the fixes suggested in the preceding pages still stand as a unique and effective roadmap for how to repair our ailing health-care system.

The question on everyone's minds is what might replace Obamacare (if anything). There are some clear indications. It appears to be a host of ideas long discussed by Republicans.

1. Repeal of Obamacare through the elimination of the individual and employer participation mandates, and dropping minimum health insurance coverage standards. This is intended to enable health insurers to offer insurance with less expensive premiums, though it is acknowledged that those policies will likely carry high deductibles and offer less coverage.

2. Use of tax credits to help make health insurance more affordable and health savings accounts (HSAs) to give Americans more flexibility and control over how their health-care dollars are spent.

3. Moving control of Medicaid away from the federal government, allowing the states more flexibility and control over how Medicaid dollars are spent.

This is a set of ideas that certainly reflects Republican values. And it may make health insurance premiums more affordable. But it is not the health-care fix that America needs. In fact, it is really just a Republican version of Obamacare—an attempt to increase the number of people who have access to health insurance. The difference is that the Republicans are making more of an effort to lower the cost of health insurance premiums.

As it has been pointed out previously in *Distracted*, though, modern health insurance is not equivalent to health-care access.

First of all, more affordable health insurance premiums are not a guarantee that health care will be affordable. The high deductibles associated with these policies may prevent many people from receiving care. In addition, the less complete coverage associated with these policies may mean that many Americans will go without the care they need or have to pay for it themselves.

As with Obamacare, this may change the health-care winners and losers, and the nature of the problems people experience, but it will not eliminate them. If you are able to purchase more affordable insurance and you are lucky enough to have health issues covered by your policy, you may be a winner. But if high deductibles keep you from accessing the care you need, or if it just so happens that your narrow coverage doesn't cover necessary care when you need it, you may lose big. Tax credits may similarly increase the affordability of health insurance for some, but the same arguments apply.

As for HSAs, it is doubtful that most Americans, especially those with lower incomes, will be able to save enough to make a significant dent in a sizable health-care bill.

And finally, giving states more control of Medicaid is clearly a mixed bag. Some states have more resources and administrative competencies than others. Once again, there will be winners and losers under such a plan. In this case, that depends on which state a patient resides in.

One of the more important lessons we can derive from the Obamacare era is that if we require the commercial health insurance industry to cover everyone, and to provide anything approaching comprehensive care, they find it difficult, by their own report, to remain profitable, or to provide insurance with affordable premiums. In other words, the commercial, for-profit insurance companies are unable to provide the comprehensive solution that America needs.

Prior to Obamacare, too many American patients suffered mightily because there were no reasonable limits on the costs of their medical care, and because they could not get access to the care they needed. Our failure then was a national disgrace. In the era of Obamacare, while many more people were able to obtain health insurance, there remained far too many people who suffered because their health-care costs were too great, and who still could not obtain the care they needed (even with insurance). This remained our national disgrace.

The standards by which the success or failure of health-care reform in America should be measured are these:

1. All patients need a firm, reasonable, and affordable cap on health-care expenditures.
2. All patients need full access to a nationally determined comprehensive basket of necessary medical goods and services.
3. All patients and medical professionals need drastic administrative and bureaucratic simplification.

If we want to make actual progress, rather than continue to push the ball around, our government must guarantee these concepts as the foundation of a health-care overhaul. The administration that accomplishes this will go down in history as national heroes. It does not appear that these Republicans will be those heroes.

Just like with Obamacare, there are still no specific limits on out-of-pocket expenses, and there is no guarantee that necessary care will be covered. And there is nothing yet to indicate whether patients or health-care professionals will be freed from today's bureaucratic nightmare. The best that can be said is that, once again, the winners and the losers may change, and the nature of the failures will likely be different, but still, a large number of Americans will continue to suffer and die at the hands of our health-care system. As it was in the years prior to Obamacare, and as it was in the era of Obamacare, it is most likely that health care will continue to be a source of national disgrace, and another opportunity to fix what is broken will be wasted.

Index